Being and Well-Being

BEING and WELL-BEING

Health and the
Working Bodies of Silicon Valley

Though it recognizes the strain work has on bodies it does not criticize or try to explain why they act (at least not from an anti capitalist perspective). = it could explore this negative impact more

↓
B Foucault?/Marx? - production for who?

J. A. ENGLISH-LUECK

STANFORD UNIVERSITY PRESS

Stanford, California

Stanford University Press
Stanford, California

Library of Congress Cataloging-in-Publication Data

English-Lueck, J. A. (June Anne).
   Being and well-being : health and the working bodies of Silicon
Valley / J. A. English-Lueck.
       p. cm.
   Includes bibliographical references.
   ISBN 978-0-8047-7157-3 (cloth : alk. paper) —
   ISBN 978-0-8047-7158-0 (pbk. : alk. paper)
       1. LHealth behavior—California—Santa Clara Valley (Santa Clara
County).   2. Health attitudes—California—Santa Clara Valley
(Santa Clara County).   3. Public health—Anthropological aspects—
California—Santa Clara Valley (Santa Clara County).   4. Employees—
Health and hygiene—California—Santa Clara Valley (Santa Clara
County).   5. Work—Health aspects—California—Santa Clara Valley
(Santa Clara County).   I. Title.
RA776.9.E54   2010
362.109794'73—dc22

                                                            2010011324

Printed in the United States of America on acid-free, archival-
quality paper

Typeset at Stanford University Press in 10.5/15 Minion

*To Paul James Bohannan, my mother and my father, as the Tiv would say;
and to my brothers and sisters at the Institute for the Future*

Contents

[Handwritten annotation: explores how the conditions + customs of Silicon Valley as 'place' construct an embodied understanding of the body as adaptable subject]

Preface and Acknowledgments

Embodying Ethnography

The data for this book is drawn from more than fifteen years of study in Silicon Valley through diverse ethnographic projects, collectively called the Silicon Valley Cultures Project.[1] Actual ethnographic studies in the Silicon Valley Cultures Project include both small focused projects and large-scale ethnographic investigations. The first of the large projects, funded by the National Science Foundation, examined the interplay of work, identity, and community in Silicon Valley with multiple observations and interviews of 175 workers in the late 1990s (see English-Lueck 2002). How people lived in multiple social networks was a large part of that story. Led by myself, Charles Darrah, and James M. Freeman, our team of ethnographers, including Lori Burgman, Jason Silz, and Joe Hertzbach, talked to these workers about their careers and work lives, and mapped their physical work spaces at home and in companies. We also mapped slices of their social lives, knowing that relational networks play a central part in shaping the lives of Silicon Valley residents and sojourners (Saxenian 2006; Haveman and Khaire 2006, 278; Darrah 2007, 267).

Darrah, Freeman, and I spent another twenty-five hundred hours in deeply ethnographic participatory observations of fourteen middle-class working families at the cusp of the century, funded by the Alfred P. Sloan Foundation (Darrah, Freeman, and English-Lueck 2007). These large projects had been based primarily around scientific or policy questions; other undertakings were more explicitly applied. For example, in one project, the Santa Clara County Office of Education commissioned me and a group of San Jose State students to investigate informal learning among thirty-two of Silicon Valley's adolescents and their mentors (English-Lueck et al. 2003). San Jose State University students who worked on that project included Ryan Amaro, Ofelia Badia-Pinero, Kelly Boyle, Yen Do, Kelly Fox, Rosanna Mutia, Guillermo Narvaez, Barbara Redman-White, Layna Salzman, Sheri Swiger, and Sabrina Valade.

The Institute for the Future, a nonprofit think tank located in Palo Alto, was my major partner in generating ideas and collecting data for this book. Three relevant projects, among many others, grew out of this relationship. Researchers at the institute, Charles Darrah, and I explored the role of networks in shaping the choices, reflections, and rationalizations of digitally savvy youth. With the help of Marlene Elwell, Benjamin Dubois, and Mary McCuistion, we collected information on the social networks of twenty key individuals, ranging from their teens to their mid-twenties, located in Silicon Valley, Finland, Sweden, Japan, and Great Britain. Each of these people became a central hub. We observed and interviewed members of their personal and professional networks and closely examined the relationships, activities, places, technologies, and rhythms relevant to their lives (Gorbis et al. 2001). BRICs—another ethnographically based project—is an ongoing examination of family life. It is an open-ended five-year study of forty-seven families—in Brazil, Russia, India, China, and transnational Silicon Valley. The team—Rod Falcon, Marina Gorbis, Lyn Jeffery, Mani Pande, Andrea Saveri, and Kathi Vian—worked with me and cultural psychologist Adriana Manago. They created a method of "bottom-up forecasting," an ethnographic approach that detects changes in everyday life and anticipates their intended and unintended consequences (Falcon et al. 2006).

Many stories in this book are drawn directly from a project I did jointly with the Institute for the Future. Typically, medical forecasting is directed toward the delivery of health care services, rather than the experience of well-being and illness itself. Scenario building is based on economic trends, rather than broader contexts of everyday life. Pioneering bottom-up forecasting, the Health Horizons team—Rod Falcon, Leah Spalding, Lyn Jeffery, and students James Battle, Leah Cook, Erika Jackson, and Mary McCuistion—and I explored the "Personal Health Ecologies" of more than fifty people in the San Francisco Bay Area (Falcon and Spalding 2004). This multiyear project used a variety of tools to explore how people understand and experience the management of their health, not in a narrow sense of biomedical health care but in a broader perspective that embraced facets often excluded from analysis—beauty, well-being, workplace fatigue, and mutual support. We mapped their networks, seeking to understand who helped convey and interpret health information and who was consulted in decision-making. In addition to two focus groups, we went into people's homes and photographed the artifacts and spaces they identified as relevant to their pursuit of well-being, as well as the objects and places they identified as "unhealthy." In the first years of the study, the net was cast broadly to capture people in a range of ages and states of health. In 2004 the focus was narrowed to people at risk or diagnosed with coronary artery disease or diabetes.

In 2007, a group of students—Richard Alvarado, Erin Dunham, Louise Ly, Brianna Musa, Vincent Navarro, Michelle Nero, Krsni Watkins—and I continued to explore the personal health ecologies of eighteen more workers, eighteen to thirty-five, who were developing strategies for juggling work, family, and health. We observed and talked to practitioners of complementary/alternative medicine and women's health care, as they shared their observations about the bodies of Silicon Valley. Standing in a *qigong* studio, smelling the herbal mixtures from traditional Chinese medicine, I was brought back to my deeply participatory fieldwork among alternative health practitioners and midwives decades ago (English-Lueck 1990). I went to prediabetes and diabetes clinics and weight management events, not only to understand the people I was researching but also to manage my own health issues, since I am one of those 53 percent of knowledge workers in Silicon Valley who are overweight. I took clinics in ChiRunning and ChiWalking so that I could feel, in my own body, the experience of my informants and understand their struggle to match biomedical numbers to internally sensed states of well-being. My fieldwork career had come full circle.

No one project forms the basis of this work, but the previously mentioned projects were created or reanalyzed with the work/health connection in mind. Not all the people whose stories are used in this book are in the high-technology workforce so often identified with Silicon Valley. Yet, their workplaces include iconic organizations such as Adobe, Apple, Cisco Systems, Fairchild Semiconductors, Hewlett-Packard, Google, Lockheed, Pixar Animation Studios, and Yahoo! Other workers are employed by universities, hospitals, nonprofit organizations, small businesses, and start-ups in the region.

This book is organized around productivity, health beliefs, and practices and embodied identities as they are experienced by different age groups. Children, adolescents, younger and older adult workers, and the postretirement elderly experience the quest for productivity and the remaking of their bodies quite differently. So while the thrust of the book explores the link between productivity and the remaking of self, the overall arc is developmental, ranging from older adults who pioneered the health culture of Silicon Valley to the children who grew up in it. Field data is recent enough that most people are still in the age cohort in which they were studied, although as many as ten years may have passed. Each person's story is told at the age I observed them.

Observations of the children of dual-career families, Silicon Valley's digital youth, and the informal learning networks among high school students build the picture for young people in this book. Interviews and observations of workers imbedded in families and communities, and personal health ecologies for people in their mid-twenties through their forties form the basis for understanding the situation of the core workforce. Many of the parents studied in the dual-career family observations as well as the people whose personal health ecologies we collected were from the cohort born after World War II, ages forty-five through sixty-five. Often they had developed chronic conditions that complicated their stories as workers or family members. Sometimes, it was the presence of such a condition that led us to them. Narratives of chronic illness dominate my sample of people in their retirement years. Such problems are not always present among those over sixty-five, but a consciousness of potential ills is never far away, even among the healthy. The intermittent flirtation with work, and the lurking, near-constant consciousness of illness, makes the story of the elderly in Silicon Valley quite different from that of their younger counterparts.

I would like to acknowledge the hard work and support of my friends, students, and colleagues at San Jose State University and the Institute for the Future. The best ideas in this book are undoubtedly theirs, and I appreciate their generosity in letting me weave them together. Paul Bohannan, my late mentor, left me with a legacy of insights that reverberate throughout these pages. I have special gratitude toward Ruhama Veltfort, my stalwart editor, who directed her writer's eye to my professorial voice. My family—Karl Lueck, Eilene Lueck, Miriam Lueck Avery, and Christopher Avery—sustain and nourish me at every turn. Karl always supplies the right word; Eilene expounds the most informative interpretations of anime. Anthropologists Miriam and Chris combine theoretical discussions and family dinners in ways to delight the heart and inspire the mind.

Prologue—Clare's Hands

Clare Washington is a fifty-year-old product lead, an engineering manager for an innovative computer company, working on the integration of software with the operating systems of laptop devices. She "rides herd on people . . . tracks the tasks, the deliverables" answering only to the manager of product managers. Clare's road to high-technology work was circuitous, as she explored her identity and molded her own beliefs through different kinds of employment.

Born after World War II, she trained to be an English teacher, largely so she could relocate to the West Coast. She worked her way through college as a secretary, learning skills that directly support her current managerial work. After attending a college nestled in the countercultural communities of Oregon, she became a practitioner of *shiatsu*, a Japanese technique of body work—that itself draws on **kanpo** (**traditional Chinese medicine**) and Western traditions—to balance bodily functions. Her hospice work in Oregon paved the way for Clare to move to the San Francisco Bay Area. A lesbian activist, she worked with patients with HIV until too many of her own friends were dying. "I had death in my professional life and death in my personal life, and it was just too much." She bought a house-cleaning business, which gave her the flexibility to be "present for my friends who were dying."

Clare's introduction to the high-tech world began in customer service. She then took management courses on work styles; she went to Toastmasters to hone her communication skills. She earned an M.A. in human resources and organizational development. She views herself as "a planner," and built on that foundation. She continues to define herself as one who has "a route in my head. I am going to do this, then this, then this! . . . I'm the kind of person that likes to make dates."

She consciously built a network of politically and socially compatible people, who "operate similarly in the world" and also share an "experience of repression in the world." These people came from working-class families or had a **GLBTQ** affiliation. Gay Pride month is a time of community action and activity. She continues to explore her spirituality, creating sacred places in her house or finding them at the beach.

Her office is outfitted with the latest ergonomic devices, positioned to fit her body perfectly. In front of her are bottles of pills—antacids for stomach pain and blue-green algae for energy. She has a mirror, which allows her to see behind her back, and brings her office into harmonious *feng shui*, an East Asian practice of arranging architecture and objects to harmonize energies. In her office is a statue of the Hindu deity **Ganesha**, the remover of obstacles, "good for a project manager."

She knows her work is physically demanding. She wakes up in the middle of the night thinking about work, and about the burden of "working long hours." Clare does not like asking a coworker, who is a single father, to come in at 1:30 A.M. to do testing for a few hours, but "I need him to do that." She is upset thinking about his two children, ages eleven and fifteen, home alone. She suspects there is alcoholism and drug abuse all around her, but no one talks about it.

Work has had a huge impact on her own life. Clare had once worked on what was at that time a relatively new kind of personal digital assistant. Her team had developed a fifteen-ounce handheld device, later abandoned by the company, that, ironically, Clare herself could not hold. Clare had developed severe **carpal tunnel**. Later, at her home, Clare told me about the changes that had taken place because of her disability. Once she camped with her friends; she does so no longer. Once she had been an avid reader of novels, now she reads only magazines. She does not surf the web for pleasure, but looks at her hands, saying, "I really can't justify using them for my personal pleasure when I need to save them for work." She opens her drawer and shows me the prototype for the PDA, the one she cannot hold. She holds up her hands, stares intently at them and says, "I save these for [my company]."

1   Embodying Place

There's no telling
What's on the mind
Of the bony
   Character in plaid
Workcoat & glasses
   Carrying lunch
   Stalking and Bouncing
   Slowly to his job
—Kerouac 1995, "11th Chorus," 12

The Tectonic 2.5

The year is 2005. The Silicon Valley is beginning to come back from the dot-com bust of 2001. Each January, Joint Venture Silicon Valley Network, a public private partnership, issues an annual index assessing the business and social challenges of the previous year. Because I gather people's stories as a cultural anthropologist, I relish the chance to study the numeric data gathered by Collaborative Economics from diverse governmental and private databases. Sitting in my office, glued to the screen scanning the downloaded file of the index, I scroll to the table of contents. I read, "Valley Productivity Rises to 2.5 Times National Average." I sit there, stunned, feeling as if I were enduring some sort of conceptual earthquake. How is this remarkable figure accomplished? I think of Clare's hands. I turn to page twenty and continue to read, "In 2004, the region's value added of $224,200 per employee is more than two-and-half times U.S. value added per employee of $85,800" (Henton et al. 2005). Value-added, a sacred phrase in the **new economy**, is a measure of compensation and profit, estimated by regional gross domestic product, per employee, a short-hand for worker contribution to productivity. I check to make sure that all employees, including **temporary workers**, are included, and so it appears. Such value-added can be created and diminished rapidly by technologically enhanced productivity and shifts in market value. Having observed and talked to hundreds of workers, however, I know it is also the result of intense effort, long hours coupled with bursts of creativity. In the years following that watershed event, although the number fluctuates along with the troubles of the national economy, Silicon Valley's per capita productivity has continued to rise, surpassing even the boom years at the turn of the century (Henton et al. 2008, 14). After encountering that statistic, I felt, in addition to empathic exhaustion, compelled to mine my ethnographic data systematically to examine the relationship of work and health in Silicon Valley.

Everyday life is illuminated by blending together social creativity, bodily discipline, **medical pluralism,** and work morality. Recurrent themes emerge as we examine the stories of **embodied** lives in Silicon Valley.

First, *place matters.* The particular setting of Silicon Valley shapes the larger chronicle. While some aspects of the region's culture are shared with that of other Americans, and immigrant homelands, other facets are distinct. Silicon Valley shares its history with the rest of California and the San Francisco Bay Area. It does, however, distinguish itself as a center of technological development. The associated values of pragmatic efficiency shape its work, family, and **health cultures**. Policies, set at the national and state level, establish different conditions to which people must adapt. The historical development of particular regions, such as the San Francisco Bay Area, shapes the tools people can access to make those accommodations. Moreover, as a model and a metaphor for a technological future, Silicon Valley sends a potent iconic message for the rest of the United States, and the world.

Second, the *ethos* of experimentation, both scientific and **countercultural**, catalyzes the creation of novel cultural practices. The self becomes a project, subject to endless tinkering. Can those bodily experiments, dietary or pharmaceutical, lead to greater productivity?

- Third, Silicon Valley's _cultural complexity_—as people migrate, interact, and borrow—creates a distinctive form of medical pluralism. Work, family, and health beliefs and practices flow from many cultural origins. The multiple beliefs and practices around bodily care, derived from many parts of the world, are interlaced with alternative healing modalities that are themselves global in origin. Chinese herbs are sold in Latino **botánicas.** Clients can take holistic yoga classes at a local gym while simultaneously visiting Indian-trained **Ayurvedic** practitioners straight from South Asia for advice on diet.

- Fourth, people are _restaging the life course._ **Life staging**—dependent child, productive adult, and inactive elder—is being rethought as the sequence of work becomes more unpredictable and the lines of age-related disease are being redrawn. Children are drawn into productive work, and retirement from employment may not be practical for people over sixty. Children are diagnosed with what was once considered "adult-onset" **diabetes,** and fifty-year-old amateur athletes resist the specter of inevitable chronic disease.

- Finally, _structural changes in the political economy_ drive people into greater individuation, as they must rely on themselves to manage their own educational, career, financial, and health care decisions, with less support from outside institutions. The dual processes of work **intensification** and the reorientation of health care from institution to individual are taking place all over the world. Employment is more contingent and more unpredictable. Those left standing must work more intensely. The drive for productivity dominates the lives of Silicon Valley workers, and allows them to _feel_ capitalism intimately in their everyday lives.

These five topics—Silicon Valley's geographic distinctiveness; rampant experimentation; cultural complexity; life restaging; and economic individuation—structure our discussions.

We often look at work, especially the "new" work of the twenty-first century, as if it were part of an ethereal global landscape where digital flows of information transform life (see Hakken 1993). Work, particularly knowledge work, is not confined to particular hours or places; work is not a sealed domain, but one that intertwines with the rest of life. The work that produces this economy is done by real flesh and blood men and women; life on this side of the screen is not abstract but *embodied*. Particularly in a place that has become iconic for the high-technology global economy—a bellwether for the rest of the United States—knowing that actual people embody that labor transforms the way we think of knowledge workers. The region's high-tech economy is volatile, producing booms and busts that are experienced as intense physical episodic and daily stress. The high-tech industry has also left a dystopian environmental legacy. **Clean rooms,** the birthplace of integrated circuits, are kept pristine for the circuits, not for the people. Project-based work has expanded to include a variety of life practices. Relationships, identities, and health states become *projects* in everyday practice, to be **augmented** by technology. The work practices and **pragmatism** that underlie the drive for productivity enhance human integration with devices and technologies, including medical technologies. At the same time, a deeply romantic attitude toward nature pervades **complementary and alternative medicine (CAM)** so that people who use this approach simultaneously embrace and revile technology. Individuals both use and doubt technologies, but in different contexts in their lives.

There has been a tangible change in the intensity of activities faced by workers that we once would have identified as middle-class (Gershuny 2005, 309). Mastering technologies, responding to work pressures, meeting the increasingly individuated obligations of parenthood, and simply understanding what to buy in the grocery store to make sure the daily meals are healthful, reshape everyday life (Darrah 2007; Darrah, Freeman, and English-Lueck 2007). Family, as well, is not experienced in the abstract, but in the bodies of its members. Indeed, evidence indicates that busyness in the family, especially in families with small children, curtails time for physical exercise, and intensification at work and home leads to less healthful food choices (Allen and Armstrong 2006). Staying healthy becomes another set of activities to squeeze into a hectic life.

The people—workers and family members—in Silicon Valley experiment on themselves using both rational scientific **biomedical** and nonbiomedical alternative practices. Silicon Valley is part of Northern Californian and the larger Bay Area experimental counterculture. Catholic, feminist,

Zen, and Hindu shrines rest next to engineering diagrams in corporate cubicles. Alternative medical notions and genetic information are used side-by-side with little concern that these practices harness different types of medical logic. In the early years of the twenty-first century, between 35 and 40 percent of Silicon Valley's population is foreign born. This statistic masks the deeper complexity of cultural borrowing, mixing, and editing as people dynamically define and categorize each other, in the domains of both work and health practices. Each of these activities is experienced differently across the life course.

By understanding that family, health, and work are all *embodied* experiences, we can come to see that these are not several separate stories, but a single narrative with intertwining plotlines. We will explore this grand story, from the perspective of people who nurture, hurt, and toil in a region that is both distinctive—even other silicon places do not have Silicon Valley's particular profile—and strangely familiar. The face of the United States is changing. Economic and social interconnections with the rest of the world are becoming part of Middle America. The integration of technology into everyday life is happening in Kansas City as well as San Francisco. The changes in the institutions and practices of work and health are easily seen in Silicon Valley—early adopters of the new economy—but such alterations are not unique to it.

[handwritten margin note: Suggesting neolib effects on embodied experiences of life might be visible here first?]

Geographies of Work and Health

Silicon Valley reflects larger geographies of work and health. The United States is the federal political unit in which policy, the structures of insurance law, and the unique institutions of employer-based health care have evolved. Immigration policy is enacted at the national level, moderating the flow of sojourners and new citizens, who bring new work and health cultures with them. Institutions such as Medicare and Medicaid are federal programs providing health care. Individual states also fund care and add yet another layer of bureaucracy and policy. Health care is distributed unequally, as is the disposal and clean up of industrial toxins; this geography of inequality is inscribed on worker bodies. Some live in healthful places and can afford to enhance themselves beyond being merely well, and others struggle to eat properly and find treatment outside of hospital emergency rooms. In California, the intricacy of cultural relations has complicated access to resources while also enriching the pool of potential health practices.

The people of Santa Clara and San Mateo counties, the governmental entities that compose Silicon Valley, have a life span fully two and a half years beyond the national average, 80.26 years. While many counties, especially in the American South, have seen a decline in life expectancy, especially for women, this is not true for Silicon Valley (Lyons 2008; Ezzati et al. 2008). The Silicon Valley population is relatively wealthy, educated, and working on being **better than well**. They live longer, particularly as many of the elderly poor move away to lower cost of living regions.

Location is of critical importance in this ethnography, suggesting that time and place matter. A historic slice of this region in the 1930s would reveal a place repeatedly redefined by immigration from Asia and Europe, but still quite similar to the other coastal Californian agricultural towns, so compellingly described by John Steinbeck. The alchemy of change brought by the aerospace, electronics, and information technology industries, and the concomitant influx of American and international migrants, later transforms Silicon Valley and distinguishes it from neighboring regions.

The San Francisco Bay Area has historically been a conduit for cultural influx, both of immigrants and global ideas. This was already true in the nineteenth century, but the region became identified with multiculturalism and countercultural experimentation from the 1950s onward. The first ethnic studies programs were developed there (Teraguchi 2004). Emerging values of **sexual liberation** mingled with feminist politics, experimental relationships, and a discourse of **self-actualization** as the technologies of reproduction changed sexual practices in the sixties and seventies. The centrality of the region to food, health, sexual, and social countercultural movements is an essential part of our larger story. While parts of these movements may be manifest elsewhere, the density of mutually reinforcing changes in one region intensified the movement in the Bay Area. Revolutions in diet, **holistic health**, and a re-establishment of the sanctity of nature changed the culinary and medical practices of Bay Area people.

Silicon Valley, as a place, is set within other regions that have their own stories. It is part of the San Francisco Bay Area, and California, especially in its history of immigrant **ethnoscapes** and social movements. Key elements of the Silicon Valley story, the commingling of many cultures, the celebration of nature, the optimism about technology, are imbedded in the history of California, as are its social injustices and environmental injuries (Park and Pellow 2004; Starr 2005). The region played a key historic role during the nineteenth-century Gold Rush as a source of mercury, a toxic metal used in gold ore processing (Pellow and Park 2002, 34). That historic event and the expansion that followed brought waves of immigrants from Latin America and Asia, priming the "insertion of Sino-America" into California (Starr 2005, 19). As early as 1850, the San Francisco Bay Area was becoming a culturally distinct region, a gateway to the rest of the world. It is not coincidence that the people, money, and ideas for California's nineteenth-century flirtation with creating a Marxist utopia at Kaweah, in the southern Sierra Nevada, flowed from the bay. By the onset of the twentieth century, the popular culture of the day was strongly marked by "three continuing preoccupations: nature, naturalism, and bohemia." The founding of Berkeley's University of California and Palo Alto's Stanford University further promoted the notion of California as a "natural place" (ibid., 153–58).

At the same time, innovations in mining, agricultural, military, and communications technologies were establishing California as a major center of technological innovation. These impulses, romantic naturalism, and instrumental techno-optimism went hand in hand. California "was linked to the effort to discover a truth, solve a problem, make a profit, make productive use of one's time, and in the process, make the world a better and more interesting place. Open, flexible, entrepreneurial, unembarrassed by the profit motive, California emerged as a society friendly to the search for utopia through science and technology" (ibid., 247). That particular utopian effort led to the technocrats of Silicon Valley; although many inhabitants would characterize it as dystopian rather than idyllic!

Another facet of this search led from the Bohemians to the **Beats**, which included the poets Lawrence Ferlinghetti, Allen Ginsberg, Jack Kerouac, and Asian-oriented, anthropologically trained Gary Snyder. Embracing sex, experimenting with chemically induced cognition, modifying and interpreting Zen, rejecting conformist capitalism, and rebelling against the status quo, the Beats laid the literary foundation for the social movements of the 1960s (ibid., 287–88). These movements brought changes in lifestyles to embrace holistic health, ecological consciousness, and the consumption of **natural food**.

The resurgence of **American Transcendentalism**—a philosophy that celebrates nature, pragmatism, and experimentation—in the San Francisco Bay Area reoriented some of the basic philosophical principles of that tradition. Thoreau and his followers gazed toward Asia, albeit one of artistic imagination, for validation. In the twentieth century the remnants of this Orientalism were informed by a new reality. The Bay Area was inhabited by living Asians, and by people who had spent time in Asia. *Taijiquan* practitioners, yoga teachers, acupuncturists, herbalists, and aficionados of Asian cuisine proliferated, their practices ultimately augmented by websites, videos, and online recipes. Farmers' markets and new retail chains that integrated alternative and mainstream products, from **Whole Foods Market** to **Elephant Pharmacy**, had a distinct Asian flavor.

This movement, too, is utterly integrated with the origins of Silicon Valley. Communications scholar Fred Turner and journalist John Markoff each make a compelling case that seminal technocrats—from Douglas Englebart, inventor of the mouse and the graphical user interface, to the infamous **Homebrew Computer Club** participants Steve Wozniak and Steve Jobs, who founded Apple—were deeply immersed in the counterculture (Turner 2006; Markoff 2006). Digital utopianism emerged from the counterculture. Nature is exalted, but given new contexts for abstraction. Steward Brand was part of a nexus of catalysts that included anthropologist Gregory Bateson, **Merry Prankster** Ken Kesey, and technological innovators Doug Englebart and Bill English (Kirk 2007, 128). Brand advocated to NASA for a depiction of the whole earth, and used the resulting 1972 "blue marble" photograph on the cover of the *Whole Earth Catalog* (Turner 2006, 69). *Nature* extended beyond Walden Pond to embrace a systemic, cybernetic understanding of ecology. It was an imprint for a sophisticated amalgam of technology and spiritual politics. The *Whole Earth Catalog* and the *CoEvolution Quarterly* were pivotal publications in shaping the values of the digirati of the sixties and seventies, such as Steve Jobs of Apple. The centrality of the region to food, health, and sexual and social countercultural movements is an essential part of our larger story. While parts of these movements may be manifest elsewhere, the density of mutually reinforcing changes in one region intensified the movement in the Bay Area.

At the same time, an abhorrence of pollution, toxicity, and the artificiality of processed foods formed the basis for a revolution in food preferences. Cheap ethnic food was revolutionary, reflecting "whole earth" sensibilities, and rejecting mainstream food companies (Belasco 2007). Organic, community-grown food represented a return to nature that was both nostalgic and a political critique of agribusiness. It reinforced the ethic of nineteenth-century Transcendentalists, that nature is healthy. Green is clean. The rhetoric of the counterculture, while superficially communal, centered on an ideal of the uniqueness and agency of the individual. The logic of the unique person fit better with the underlying **epistemology** of the naturalistic medical systems of holistic healing than biomedicine's statistical approach. Statistical aggregation of people into epidemiological disease populations or market segments is antithetical to the revived transcendental empowerment of the individual. Natural foods, organic farming, and ethnic cuisine perfectly complemented alternative approaches to healing.

In the late nineteenth century, professional biomedicine came to dominate over the many American immigrant and **naturopathic/homeopathic** cultures of health. In the San Francisco Bay Area, the late-twentieth-century influx of immigrants and countercultural questioning of the status quo led to increased experimentation with those plural medical beliefs. Through conscious consumerism, people juggle a variety of medical body-related practices. The **modularity** that accompanied the industrial age allows practices to be merged from radically different origins. Competitive marathon running and *taiji* combine to become **ChiRunning**. Organic food can be cooked in French style with medically approved portion sizes. Prosthetics, yoga, and diet Coke can all be harnessed to maximize energy and productivity, in actions that are informed by the stories of friends and family and then replicated throughout their personal network. The actual clinical encounter between a patient and a practitioner is the narrowest strip of experience in a much wider panorama. The blended roles of patient, consumer, and augmented-self produce something new that would confuse previous generations of biomedical practitioners. The mainstreaming of global health concepts and practices coupled with the technological management of information creates a distinctive cultural pattern of doing, being, and well-being.

Ecological sensibilities combine with ethnic ingredients to create a new cuisine (ibid.). While certainly not limited to this region, San Francisco and its neighbors were seminal participants and advocates of a distinctive health culture. Production and consumption of the material culture related to those practices was an integral piece of local culture. You can go to the Café Gratitude for raw organic lunches or find numerous acupuncturists who were trained in Taiwan, or at the local American College of Traditional Chinese Medicine.

Ironically, the individuated practices of the counterculture have become the growth industries of the twenty-first century. At the turn of this century, 40 percent of American adults bought natural health alternatives, generating at least $27 billion (Eisenberg et al. 1998). Such remedies blend the modern and the traditional, appealing to the cosmopolitan consumer (Lock and Nichter and Lock 2002, 13). Wellness therapies do not just consume "foreign bodily practices" but are "also upheld as ways of remedying social and environmental illnesses" (Lau 2000, 4). They are global and moral. Reformulating the commercial products and services to make them "green" has opened up new markets and areas for expansion. Energy drinks, coffee, tea, colas, and other vehicles for the sale of caffeine provide the "drug that made the modern world possible" (Reid 2005, 15). The quest for wellness, and better than well, is hardly outside the structures of capitalism (see Photograph 1).

Silicon Valley's slice of that health culture is seen through the lens of productivity. South Bay Beat poets and Merry Pranksters dropped hallucinogenic drugs, and redirected computing science. Organic gardeners reach out to create demonstration and teaching gardens at high-tech campuses. Augmentation and self-reinvention are metaphors that apply equally well to both technology work and wellness management. It is within that context that Silicon Valley organizations are experimenting with new formulas for renegotiating the institutional relationship between work and health. In the United States, the risks of underwriting health have shifted care to employers. In Silicon Valley, continuing employer-based insurance benefits could undermine the region's productivity advantage. As a result, the companies are driven to experiment with new models of employee-centered wellness care that emphasize health and prevention, rather than expensive health care treatments (Hymel 2006b).

The Experimental Mentality

The story Silicon Valley tells about itself has been represented in many places, from exhibits at the local Tech Museum of Innovation, to scholarly works by historians and social scientists (Starr 2005; Saxenian 2006; Lee et al. 2000). Journalists and municipal politicians repeat the story until it becomes the narrative that people retell around the water cooler. While the specific details may be disputed, the story of individual ingenuity, novel capitalization, hard work, and big rewards remains constant. There is a reason that the original Palo Alto garage of Dave Packard and Bill Hewlett, the 1934 origin of the computer giant, is marked as California Historic Landmark No. 976, the birthplace of Silicon Valley (Hewlett-Packard 2008).

Although the usual story emphasizes individual prowess and success, the industrial development of the region was thoroughly intertwined with the relocation of the many defense industry contracts to California in the fifties and sixties. Over the years the San Francisco Bay Area collected national laboratories —Lawrence Berkeley, Lawrence Livermore, Sandia, NASA Ames, and the Stanford Linear Accelerator Center (SLAC)—to do big science, while generating a halo of support and spin-off organizations. Government contractors, such as Lockheed (later Lockheed Martin) and GE Tempo, set a pattern for research and development in the private sector. Stanford's Frederick Terman pioneered a new form of social organization, tightly linking prestigious university research with commercial application, nurturing and monetizing innovation. Silicon Valley's culture of individual success is built on an unspoken safety net of large institutional support. Nonetheless, the *ethos* was one of experimentation.

Part of the lore is that failure is as important as success, for it is an indicator of playing at the edge. Silicon Valley does not produce just technology, it produces **disruptive technology**. These devices change the way whole industrial sectors are framed. Vacuum tubes, transistors, integrated circuits each fundamentally transformed electronics as wholesale revolutions. The story of Silicon Valley is related as a series of disruptive technologies that begin by revolutionizing industry and employing people, while making vast amounts of profit, only to cool down as the technologies become mainstreamed. However, rather than succumbing to a terminal boom and bust cycle, Silicon Valley creates a new disruptive technology to fuel yet another cycle of economic growth and stagnation. In the 1950s the curve went up with defense, only to plateau in the 1960s. Fairchild and the "offspring" of that company, such as Intel, Advanced Micro Devices, and National Semiconductor, started a new curve by disrupting the existing electronics industry with integrated circuits.

After that peak, personal computers, associated with another garage story—Apple's Jobs and Wozniak—brought another wave of innovation. Software and the Internet brought Silicon Valley to its most intense boom, and dramatic bust (Henton 2000). As long as there is enough capital, a range of potential jobs to employ both elite professional and service workers, and a sufficiency of successful experiments to encourage further monetization, the region will thrive. When a particular technology runs its course, the region "reinvents" itself with the next new thing. After the bust of 2001, the pattern of decline differed from earlier cycles. People did not leave the region, but waited expectantly for the next technological wave. Would it be biotechnology, or bioinformatics, the marriage of biotechnology and computing? Promising, but limited in its employment potential. Already the professional and managerial class makes up 47 percent of the workforce, compared with 10 percent in the United States as a whole (U.S. Census Bureau 2006c). The broader economic health of the region depends on an ability to keep the working middle class employed. Employing geneticists will not necessarily lead to regional prosperity. Will technological applications in health hold the answer? The explosion of chronic disease and the demographic of an aging population suggest this could be an important area for future disruptive technologies.

In 2006, Al Gore appeared at the "State of the Valley" event, sponsored by Joint Venture Silicon Valley Network. The atmosphere resembled a revival meeting. Green technology had arrived in Silicon Valley. It combines enormous potential for profit, the possibility of creating economic activity that would embrace a wide range of expert and support workers, and a deeply moral mission of saving the world by intensifying efficiency. The alignment of technological optimism and romantic attachment to nature is compelling, and resonant of the region's transcendental roots. So the Valley embarks on a new chapter in its story. By 2008, eleven of the top 20 patent-generating cities in the United States were in Silicon Valley. Moreover, 8 percent of the patents in Silicon Valley were copatented outside the United States, signaling the importance of global connections. Green technology patents generated in the Valley made up 23 percent of California's patents. Investment in clean technology has been going up dramatically, nearly doubling every year since 2005 (Henton et al. 2008, 14, 17). It is one of the few industry sectors that have been robust during the global economic recession. The green technology movement links together the region's transcendental utopian impulses with pragmatic economic positioning.

Deep Medical Diversity

Ethnogenesis—the creation of new culture—is intrinsic to the **deep diversity** seen in Silicon Valley. Charles Taylor's idea of deep diversity can readily be applied to this discussion of health and well-being. Alice Water's refashioning of natural food, Gary Snyder's Zen literary fusion, and Jerry Garcia's Deadhead music formed a background for cultural experimentation that was distinct. Immigrant, sojourner, and ethnic cultures manifest and interact. Deep diversity and the concomitant **deep medical diversity** shape the anthropological artifacts of this region; I would not have detected them as easily elsewhere. The particulars of this cultural region make certain kinds of intellectual insights readily perceptible.

Taylor notes that the differences between our ancestral identities, derived from ethnicity or regional affiliation, reach deeply into the ways we act in the world. These differences are not superficial, but embodied in our very selves (Redhead 1999, 194). Deep diversity suggests that the toleration and coexistence of many forms of difference, when clustered together in a complex diverse ethnoscape, creates a wholly discrete experience of everyday life (see Elshtain 2004; English-Lueck 2002, 137; Taylor 1994, 181–84; Taylor 1993). The more differences—whether those differences are based on ancestral identity or consumer choice—the deeper the diversity. A social environment with a few ethnic and class-based differences is fundamentally different from one with dozens, or hundreds, of overlapping identity groupings where new cultural fusions abound.

While Taylor, and other political philosophers, discussed deep diversity as a template for creating governance, I consider it to be an appropriate cultural descriptor for Silicon Valley. There, work and other pragmatic values make it possible for the many forms of difference to flourish in some contexts, and in other cases to be overshadowed by the need to produce. In some situations it is important to embody Latino identity, in others, to be a materials engineer. This dance of moving elements of cultural performance from foreground to background creates malleable identities. In everyday life, identities are constantly being created, enacted, negotiated, and submerged as needed.

One set of cultural elements in this region is based on a complex stratigraphy of immigration, migration, interaction, and intermarriage. Other differences are constructed around values, behaviors, affinities, stories, and practices. Geeks, gangstas, **anime *otaku*** (fans), and Apple aficionados form foundations for other identities. These self-constructed personae may intersect with ancestral identity—many *otaku* are Asian-American—or may act separately from such identities to form new ones. These new ways of being include practices related to health—eating, moving, thinking, and feeling.

Most discussions of alternative healing distinguish the practices derived from immigrant traditions from those that come from the holistic health movement (Kaptchuk and Eisenberg 2001). The Ayurveda practiced by Indian sojourners is different from the one that evolved out of the Theosophical flirtation with India in the late nineteenth century. The latter evolved into myriad practices, including American yoga and Polarity therapy that **New Age** adherents identify with Indian medicine. The specific practices, postures, edible morsels, and massage strokes might be quite similar, but how they are integrated into everyday life differs between immigrants and new adherents. However, reinforcing this distinction leads us away from an intriguing question.

What happens when, in conditions of deep diversity, immigrant-derived medical pluralism coexists intimately with the alternative health practices that evolved in the United States? How does the experience of medical pluralism change when both kinds of alternative practice co-occur in the same neighborhoods, schools, and workplaces? Could there be a form of deep diversity that might be called deep medical diversity? This circumstance captures the complexity, the toleration, and the embodied intimacy of these global alternative practices.

Recent scholarship suggests a deep level at "which bodies are socially constructed" (Lock and Farquhar 2007, 110). If the social landscape of the region is itself deeply diverse, then the ways in which people perceive their body, their health, illnesses, and therapeutic interventions are also deeply medically plural. Deep medical diversity is characterized by borrowing concepts and practices, authenticating their cultural authority, and normalizing a wide variety of health practices.

Deep diversity is not just a dense, shifting assemblage of existing cultural categories, but reflects the agency people have in creating new combinations, making novel interpretations, and inventing avant-garde expressions. In other words, the deep diversity of the region is not a function of only migration and intermarriage but also of the experimentation. Playing with culture, with explanations of health and wellness, with new practices and postures, is also part of the region's deep medical diversity.

Silicon Valley is marked by two distinctive characteristics: the penetration of technology into the ecology of everyday life, and the less often discussed social, ethnic, and cultural diversity of the region. The first forms the context for economic growth, and the second constantly renews the regional workforce. Out of this formula, Silicon Valley develops a cheerful but fundamentally pragmatic ethic of efficiency (English-Lueck 2002). It is inefficient to exclude potentially valuable workers, so that the pursuit of success trumps the more virulent forms of social oppression.

However, I would not want to overstate the meritocracy in the region. While *searching* for a better life is hardly confined to the elite, *experiencing* a high quality of life is not necessarily for the masses. Silicon Valley's rich/poor gap continues to widen, boom or bust (Benner 2002, 210). As noted by the former mayor of San Jose, there is a bit of the Third World in every First World city (McEnery 1994, 288).

Silicon Valley is a hub of global immigration. Two shifts in immigration policy made this possible. First, the 1965 Hart-Celler Act increased the proportion of immigration from Asia, from 4 percent during the 1901–1920 period to 39 percent during the interval from 1980 to 1993. During that time, waves of ethnic Chinese Vietnamese came to the Silicon Valley region, along with other Vietnamese refugees (Freeman 1995, 32–33). The second shift came when the 1990 amendment of existing immigration law expanded the use of H1-B visas to recruit skilled workers, particularly from India and greater China (Saxenian 2006, 51–53). Some 14 percent of the science and engineering workforce in Silicon Valley is from India, and 8 percent is from China (Henton et al. 2007, 7). Between the established practice of worker importation, a California tradition harkening back to the days of mining and agricultural development, and the recruitment of skilled workers, the region was transformed into a minority majority space by the 2000 census (see Banerjee 2006).

This migration created a mélange that is only partially revealed by census categories. Nearly 2.5 million people live in Silicon Valley, which is an amalgam of Santa Clara County and parts of San Mateo, Santa Cruz, and Alameda counties. In this region:

- 40 percent are "white, non-Hispanic";
- 28 percent are from Asia (although many South Asians will not necessary so self-identify);
- 25 percent are Hispanic;
- 3 percent are African American; and
- Less than 1 percent are Native American, in spite of the fact that the Bay Area is home to one of the largest populations of urban Indians (Henton et al. 2008, 2; Ramirez 2007; Henton et al. 2009).

While 12 to 13 percent of the nation is foreign born, thirty-six percent of Silicon Valley residents were born outside the United States (Hirschman 2005, 598; Henton et al. 2008, 10; U.S. Census Bureau 2006b, 1; Henton et al. 2009). Forty-five thousand people in the San Jose–Sunnyvale–Santa Clara cities identify themselves as belonging to two or more "races." In the year 2000, 60 percent of California's mixed-race births occurred in Santa Clara County, the primary administrative unit in Silicon Valley (Stern 2005, 5). Repeatedly, these immigrants and multicultural families talk about the "tolerance" of the Valley as one of its primary assets.

The raw numbers tell only part of the story.[1] On one hand, the mixture of diverse groups is creating a cosmopolitan generation where difference is taken for granted, and even given a tightly controlled measure of celebration. These populations are connected to the rest of the world politically, socially, emotionally, and spiritually. Literally, through the global exchange of food and cuisines, people in Silicon Valley are consuming the rest of the world (Hirschman 2005). This globalization of Silicon Valley is also reflected in its health marketplace.

Shopping for Health

On the surface, it is clear that multiple cultures would imply plural medical systems as well. Chinese immigrants, and especially their parents, would want not only Chinese speaking biomedical physicians but also herbalists and acupuncturists, preferably trained in China. The scope of migration makes such pockets of cultural preference possible. Like other urban crossroads, the Silicon Valley region plays host to a number of health care traditions, playing to the diverse medical beliefs and practices of their clientele. Hindu temples and Mexican *botánicas* provision Ayurvedic practitioners and **curanderos** for Indian and Latino sojourners.

There is another layer beneath the obvious cultural pluralism. Traditions fragment, and parts move without the whole body of knowledge moving with them. Clare's use of Ganesha for spiritual fine-tuning is different from the practices of the Indian H1-B visa-holder down the corridor. She is integrating that piece of South Asian culture with many other cultural fragments of different origin. Indeed, many immigrants are more enthusiastic consumers of Western biomedicine than is Clare. Like other Indians in the United States, they use whatever tool works best for them in their medical "tool box" (Desai 2005, 431).

Complementary and alternative medicine, also known as holistic health practice, borrows parts of long-standing medical lore from ancient Asian and European traditions, and mixes those practices with contemporary popular psychology, self-help subject matter, and American Transcendental metaphysics, while placing them in a modern consumer context (English-Lueck 1990; Fuller 2005). Based on subtle and deeply subjective embodied states, these traditions emphasize balance, energy, and the agency of the individual. Energy here means not only *qi*, aura, or *prana* but also the feeling of vitality that allows people to enhance themselves (Ho 2007). That extra zest directly translates into the capacity to boost productivity and fend off exhaustion. Consumption of these alternative products, even outside of California, cuts across age groups and religious beliefs (Mears and Ellison 2000). Anthropologists associate such alternative practices as resistance to the power and control of biomedicine (Hess 2007, 469).

As we will explore in upcoming chapters, and as we saw with Clare, interaction between the technologies of biomedicine and experimentation in alternative healing is complex, situated in the particular mix of rationality and countercultural experimentation that occurs in Northern California. People create a health-related cultural pastiche, drawing on diverse traditions with different amounts of romanticism, Orientalism, pragmatism, and experimentation.

There is an obvious, but sometimes inconvenient, reality that work is not disembodied. Work with digital data is still very much linked to our physical bodies on this side of the screen. Those bodies ache, imbibe medication, and move through exercises. People are monitored using medical traditions that range from urban shamanism to the most technologically mediated forms of biomedicine. People use, understand, and rationalize their bodies drawing on many health traditions. Self-styled cyborgs, that fuse organic human bodies with information technologies, also experiment with ancient forms of meditation. Silicon Valley is situated at the global crossroads of people and capital. We should not believe, however, that all cultures in this widened medical horizon are considered equal, just because they coexist. In health, as in the workplace, power matters. Power can be manifest in material ways—defining the access to medical resources and organized care. It can also be more ethereal, as the ability to define the rules of engagement—what kinds of care are legitimate—that vary by class, culture, and age.

Restaging Life in Silicon Valley

Living, working, thriving, and struggling are experienced differently for people as they age. The demands of work and family are felt differently for thirty-year-olds establishing careers and sixty-year-olds contemplating the culturally expected stages of retirement. Similarly, health events are dramatically different over the life course, and concerns about vaccinations, child birth preparation, and hip replacements are age sensitive. Moreover, the staging of life, which is manifest in the subtle cultural expectations directed at each age group, is becoming less predictable. Changes in the economy, the nature of work, the infusion of new cultural models through immigration, and changes in the **health span**—the vitality people can reasonably expect at different ages—rework life's staging. The kinds of work expected, and available, do differ for people of different ages. For young people, opportunities to intern at NASA sit side by side with **McJobs**. Serious careers begin after schooling, but at what age is that? In an area where advanced degrees are the norm, adulthood may begin at seventeen, or thirty. Retirement can start at fifty, sixty-five or being reworked into perpetual part-time employment. In a 1999 study, surveyed corporate CEOs thought forty-three the peak age for productivity (Moen and Roehling 2005, 94). What happens to those who are fifty-three? Work patterns follow the life course imperfectly, as people move in and out of their careers. High-tech work is particularly ephemeral.

The staging of health, work, and family life by age is an important conceptual tool. However, age does not exist in a vacuum. The factors that mold each age group are situated in a historic context. Events of the day, whether that day was in 1950 or 2001, shape the cultural realities in which people live. **Cohort**[2] effect refers to the consequences of common experiences shared by a particular age set. Americans under thirty are marked by the events of September 11, 2001, and the advent of the iPhone, but they think of Civil Rights movements, the war in Vietnam, and the appearance of television in the middle twentieth century as ancient history. However, those are the events that shaped the popular culture of people born in the decade after World War II. The Korean War and World War II, and the economic and political cultures that accompanied those events, structured the expectations of their immediate elders, now in retirement. Similarly, adults now entering their forties grew up in times of recession: falling real incomes, a downsized middle-class, inflation, and the explosion of low-paying service jobs, but they knew their way around personal computers (Ortner 1998; Zemke, Raines and Filipczak 2000). They also knew that in an economic crunch corporate loyalty goes only one way (Smola and Sutton 2002). Each cohort grew up with different dominant technology, drawing on metaphors from the popular and public culture of *their* time.

However, the events outlined above are only the ones that shaped the cohorts of the United States. If you are from India, Mexico, Vietnam, China, or the island of Taiwan, your experience as a cohort is different from the person working and living next to you. The Cultural Revolution or the assassination of Indira Gandhi may be more personally and historically relevant than Reaganomics. Even what constitutes an appropriate life course is culturally shaped. A parent might ask, "Should children play, or should they study?" When does childhood end? For a well-educated Taiwanese intellectual, age thirty marks the onset of masculine adulthood according to Confucian ideals. However, if a Latino man did not take up adult duties long before thirty, his family would be gravely worried. How should you feel when you are older? Some sixty-year-olds, constantly tinkering with their bodies, buy books on **aging well** and take Zumba exercise classes, while immigrant Chinese grandparents talk about the inevitability of the machinery of the body breaking down. The changes in work and health across the life course reflect multiple cultural scripts for the staging of life.

The subtle tooling of *self* for work begins with the children. Children are not workers, but they have already begun to imagine themselves as workers. Children as young as six dream of careers. By the time they leave elementary school, they begin to adjust their dreams, putting them more in line with family realities (Moen and Roehling 2005). Those realities reflect less intergenerational class mobility than ever; children rarely migrate from their parents' class status (Auerhahn et al. 2007, 12). These young people are **digital natives**, who think of email as an archaic technology, something one uses to email thank-you notes to Grandma. They think of texting and instant messaging with their friends as intimate forms of communication (Benko and Weisberg 2007, 181; see also Johanson 2007, 179). Nonetheless, young people take work very seriously indeed (Smola and Sutton 2002, 367). They see their parents work, with vastly varying awareness of what they do. Some teens in Silicon Valley can barely articulate what their parents do for a living, while others are virtual apprentices. They are the recipients of the largess of work when parents are employed, and the stresses of unemployment when they are not.

As young people move into the long productive years of adulthood, they face a world different from their parents. The cultural expectations for when to marry, work, and have children are changing. In the last decade of the twentieth century there has been a 71 percent increase of the number of unmarried couples living together, and childbirth has been delayed. A mother's age at childbirth has gone up 2.7 years in the last thirty (Moen and Roehling 2005, 27–65). The old predictable work world of nine to five is no longer the norm. Shift work is more common, and flexible time makes planning the articulation of work and family even less predictable. Small companies, start-ups, and spin-offs, so essential in the Silicon Valley economy, are particularly difficult for working women, as this is a culture "defined by displays of masculinity and technical prowess" and expectations of heroic work effort (Baron et al. 2007, 51). Asking for flexibility, a tool used for work-life balance, is stigmatized, particularly for men (Benko and Weisberg 2007, 64). Adult workers are not homogeneous, and people just entering the workforce, in their twenties, have significantly different ways of interacting with technology and each other (ibid., 48, 181). Silicon Valley's technology workforce is aging. The average Cisco employee is now forty (Hymel 2006a). These children of less stable households watched their obsessed parents give their all to work and pay the price for it. They are more skeptical about the relationship of employer to employee.

The relationship of work and life itself has undergone a fundamental shift. The separation of these domains was a historically brief time period, primarily during the postwar period in which men were breadwinners and spouses stayed at home. Currently, only 17 percent of the population have stay-at home mothers and working fathers in the same household (Benko and Weisberg 2007, 2).

Decline in real wages, coupled with the women's movement, led to more dual career households within the middle class. The shifting nature of work, increasingly technologically mediated, meant that work could go where technology could go—and it went into households. Work, parenting, and consumption all became more intense, with more activities and expectations packed into each moment. Life became busier. Work, especially portable knowledge work, has also extensified, become more widely distributed across time and space (Jarvis and Pratt 2006). The United States "outpaces" the rest of the world in work week hours (Levine 2005, 358). Some scholars, such as sociologists Robinson and Godbey, argue that there is only a perception of feeling rushed, that there really is not less time available (Robinson and Godbey 2005, 419). Yet, if you reframe busyness not as a function of hours in the day but of activities in those hours, you can see busyness in a different light (Darrah, Freeman, and English-Lueck 2007).

Family and work trends in the United States make the career paths of individuals less certain, more tenuous, and increasingly mismatched (Benko and Weisberg 2007, 34). The ideal model of the life course of work, like the idea of the stay-at-home mother, is becoming less reflective of lived reality. Education, career entry, longevity of tenure in a position, and retirement no later than sixty-five, do not really define a predictable middle-class "career ladder," but rather a career lattice, in which a clear path up is not defined and people move across jobs and in and out of work (Moen and Roehling 2005; Benko and Weisberg 2007).

Even in the best of economic times, the nature of high-technology work both lends itself to mental health and works against it. The apparent autonomy of working on project time is a double-edged sword. In project time, life is organized around the completion of particular projects, out of sync with bodily time. While there is a discourse of self-management in the work, there are many forms of control exerted on individual workers to increase their productivity. These "entrepreneurs of their careers" were encouraged to push themselves (see Shih 2004, 231–37). Workers are shifted from project to project to maximize their output, placing them in a constant state of intensification.

In the early 1990s workers told us how they could experience the entire life cycle of a project, from joyous and relaxed creation to intensified deadline rush. However, as work intensified, often with pressure from investors, they would work on multiple projects, so that they experienced the compacted final rush as their enduring daily experience. Controlling the overall allocation of work was not very autonomous at all! In his late 1980s social psychological research on work stress, Karasek noted that exhaustion, "feeling stressed," and experiencing temporal pressure related to milder stress-related symptoms. Those who had less autonomy in their work felt a keener depression. On a day-to-day basis, "low decision latitude" was a significant factor in mental and physical health. He postulated that professionals and managers had such autonomy. However, in his study of a "new economy" plant in Fremont, he found that work was packed in and intensified, and that the rule of the day was "management by stress" (Karasek 1990, 9, 49–59).

Engineering work itself became more routinized over the following years, involving less spontaneity and eroding the experience of autonomy. Even though 62 percent of Silicon Valley workers, and 70 percent of technology workers, view their work as "creative," they are practicing this creativity within economic contexts that exert significant pressures (see Henton et al. 2006, 4). Deciding when to do each project is out of the hands of even the most creative worker. When layoffs occur, each remaining worker is subject to sudden intensification, a state that erodes the joys of creative work.

Intensely Productive

The very language of work and work practice modalities shape the way people "work on themselves." There is a morality to this connection between productivity and identity that shapes what is valued. Art, music, religion, and family roles are refashioned and then swept into work to service productivity. This recrafting resembles the way *suzhi* has been used in China to link work discipline, consumerism, and social behavior into a morality that promotes the qualities desired by the state. Adult workers function in a multicultural workplace, send their children to schools marked by deep diversity, and practice medical pluralism. They also live in a stressful world in which bodily discipline, intensification, and dysfunction are part of the theatricality of work. They use food, depressants, and stimulants to modify their sense of vitality. Selective adherence to medical regimes adds an additional element of control, one in which the morality of work is a key component. Trainers, **coaches**, and the person's networks become players in shaping what choices will be made and how those choices will be implemented.

Health is inextricably linked to productivity, not only in the profitability of the company, saving on health care costs, but in how the bodies of production are experiencing health. Work and health in America are bundled together in a set of values in which power is placed in different and often contradictory places. First, the primacy of work, a form of work ethic, prompts how I use my body. Work is a motivation, a rationalization, and a structure of power to be invoked in making health decisions. When we think about Clare's hands, we understand she is making a moral statement, clarifying that she is willingly subjugating her individual needs to the needs of her employer. This is exactly what is meant by the political economic pattern of individuation, placing the burden of responsibility on individual workers. Individuals need to produce, or at least be seen trying to produce.

Work intensification creates the conditions in which people try that much harder to be productive. Families are often at the center of this strategy; they collectively weather the onslaughts of economic, workplace-driven, and health-related crises. Family members, friends, and coworkers can create a buffer against work stress, just as they can create stresses of their own (Ducharme and Martin 2000, 224–27). In our ethnographic research on health networks, coworkers are a vital support for changing health behaviors and disseminating and vetting information, for either good or ill.

In this book, our discussion of the work and health in Silicon Valley must be couched in both macropolitical and micropolitical discussions. The bodies of Silicon Valley workers, their children and their aging parents, live in a

particular setting, an icon of late capitalism. With its technological innovation, emphasis on problem-solving, and structures selected for rapid flexible
change, twenty-first-century workers live every day with a particular kind
of work discipline (see Martin 1994). In this discipline, individuals bear the
burden of productivity. They bear responsibility for adapting to potential
sudden deskilling and retooling themselves to fit the new circumstances. It is
within this particular context that we want to understand the embodiment
of work and the range of cultural experiments that surround it.

Thinking through the Body

Theoretical tools in anthropology and the social sciences make it possible to ask the questions this book explores. In our explorations of the
medical beliefs and practices of other cultures it has been awkward to map
non-Cartesian conceptions of self onto the categories of social scientific
Cartesian dualism practiced in Europe, North America, and the antipodes.
It is difficult to talk about self without falling into the default categories of
body, mind, and spirit, reifying the divisions between them. Anthropologist
Andrew Orta notes this dilemma in his work on Aymara in the Bolivian
altiplano, as do ethnographers of Chinese medicine Farquhar and Zhang
(Orta 2000; Farquhar 1994; Zhang 2007). It is difficult for anthropologists
trained in rationalist tradition to convey a cultural understanding of the
body in which the dualist ideas of René Descartes never took root.

Working in regions of California where multiple frames of reference
are prevalent, including that of Chinese medicine, I also find it awkward
to force my informants' more integrated sense of self into distinct spheres
of abstract mind and concrete body. Those pigeonholes are losing ground,
both in the framing schema of globalized Silicon Valley, and in the thinking
of anthropologists themselves.

Anthropology is discovering the body.[3] Anthropology, like other academic disciplines, is a deeply verbal activity. Our words and our informants' words dominate our thinking (Orta 2000). The phenomenological
concepts of Merleau-Ponty posit that the world is not a projection of mind,
but that the body and the world are actively engaged in reconstructing exis-

tence together (Herzfeld 2001, 240). Although epistemological debates rage, neuroscientists such as Antonio Damasio counter Descartes by arguing that "the mind is embodied, in the full sense of the term, not just **embrained**" (James and Hockey 2007, 44–55). The "strange invention of an outside world" takes us into a realm of abstraction in which we do not actually live in the world, and our bodies do not matter (Gallagher 2005, 68). Our senses do matter and the way in which we experience and interpret sensory information is deeply subject to culture. Pierre Bourdieu took this phenomenological approach, and reformulated a concept of Marcel Mauss and gave us *habitus*, which refers to an assemblage of feelings, thoughts, tastes, and bodily postures that are structured by power, and in turn structure systems of power (Damasio 1994, 118; Latour 2007; Scheper-Hughes 2007, 461). Social power influences how these habitual states are structured and experienced. In many ways Bourdieu's concept of *habitus* is very similar to *ethos,* a term set forward by Ruth Benedict and Gregory Bateson. Gregory Bateson suggested a similarly embodied socialized psyche in *Naven,* calling it *ethos* (Bourdieu 1998, 7; Reed-Danahay 2005, 107). Bourdieu, however, places *ethos* in complex societies, linking bodily dispositions with power structures—such as class and gender—making the concepts suitable for thinking about the postcolonial planet.

Medical anthropology in particular is at the forefront of rethinking the cultures of the body, emphasizing the sense-making we humans do with the information of our senses (Bourdieu 1977, 76–87). Placing embodiment in the center of our analytical framework renews the emphasis on everyday practice and experience. Grand cultural events—such as festivals rife with symbolic images—are the favored field sites of interpretive anthropologists. When viewed as embodied culture, they are no more important than a placid day in the cubicle. Instead of embracing the abstract surety of symbols, medical anthropologists are exploring the metaphors people use to mold their frames of reference, practices, and stories. Metaphors are more amorphous than symbols, and meaning is more malleable to those who embody them (Reed-Danahay 2005, 102–7). For example, political and economic structures create metaphors that structure how people talk about their bodies. Emily Martin, in her medical anthropology classic *Flexible*

Bodies, suggests that the framework of flexibility, which is intrinsic to the workings of the new economy, created a metaphor that changes the way we understand our own bodies' immune system (Martin 1994). Before the shift in work logic, people drew on metaphors of the Cold War in which soldier-antibodies fought disease. People had thought they could "train" their immune systems to respond to the new disease environment (Reischer and Koo 2004, 307). Martin made apparent the metaphorical connection between work practices and medical explanations. Similarly, in *Bipolar Expeditions*, Martin demonstrates that the cultural affinity for *mania*, as opposed to the problematic depressive portion of bipolar disorder, resonates with postindustrial capitalism. Entrepreneurship and creativity are manic states to be valued and cultivated (2007, 257).

Thomas Csordas in particular has brought embodiment to the attention of medical anthropologists, calling the body not the "object" of culture "but an integral part of the perceiving subject" (Herzfeld 2001, 242). Influenced by Merleau-Ponty and Bourdieu, he suggests that "the body is in the world from the start" (van Wolputte 2004, 257–60). Emotions are experienced through the body, social interactions happen between bodies, and the empathy we experience is based on our extension of bodily self. While we may construct cognitive categories through which we understand the world, the world has not gone away. Our bodies are part of that world (Csordas 1990, 5, 36). Our bodies act on the world as agents (ibid., 38). This rediscovery of the body does not mean that anthropologists have forgotten about other social agencies and structures. On one level, the political economy of globalization has a direct impact on the health and welfare of those bodies. Sometimes the macropolitical connection is stunningly obvious, such as in Paul Farmer's exposition of the epidemiology of poverty (Lock and Farquhar 2007).

Twenty-first-century social problems and economic practices are providing new frameworks and metaphors. Along with the rediscovery of the body, food is becoming a central focus for macropolitical and micropolitical analysis (Farmer 2005). The politics of corn, corn syrup additives, and corn-based fuel tell us about the broad strokes of global economy and the power to shape food policy. At another level, the micropolitics of the consumption of commercial corn chips, tortillas, and polenta reveal aspects of eating *habitus*, that subtle shaping of tastes and class.

In the last twenty years, new ways of looking at human experience in anthropology and the other social sciences have opened up interesting places to explore. Debates about how best to understand human culture led anthropologists to look at public culture, and to personal everyday experience. Is culture really relevant anymore, or is it only a placeholder for the constantly morphing identities of people who happen to connect? How do anthropologists understand difference, and, perhaps more pertinently, how do the people themselves understand the distinctions they create and enact? Does a close reading of discourse—what people say and how they represent themselves—best reveal the hidden social relationships of power? Is there more to human experience than abstract structure, symbol, and power? The rediscovery of the body, as the place where human experience resides, and lives in a larger physical world of organisms and objects reminds us, as scholars of humanity, that the intellectual categories we create are not more real than our material selves, although the abstractions may shape how we think and act. Anthropology has rediscovered that the body, as it eats, sleeps, and feels a twinge of pain between the shoulder blades, is a prime portal into the rest of human experience.

Just as anthropologists are finding their bodies, they are also struggling with a redefinition of cultural experience. We had long ago abandoned the rather unsophisticated idea that each person resides in one of a limited pool of containers, that person's culture. Culture is more elastic, more active, and more prone to tinkering than many of our anthropological ancestors envisioned. Moreover, the kinds of cultural exchange possible in the mediated twenty-first century make any notion based on isolation deeply problematical. Globalization in its myriad forms not only changes the way people of different cultures interact; it has also changed the way anthropologists think about that interaction. This book may be set in Silicon Valley, and people themselves reference a Silicon Valley "culture," but a critical part of the regional adaptation is that diverse ways of thinking, creating family, working, and healing are the quotidian modus operandi, the way people live every day. We need to think through the problem of being an embodied worker of the twenty-first century, understanding that ways of working, giving care, and being well are being informed by the recombinant DNA of globalization.

Mapping the Body of the Book

As mentioned earlier, this book segregates the experiences of people based on their age cohorts. People reveal the larger social picture of their lives through "**illness narratives**," stories about their experiences with health, and its absence. This approach is part of an anthropological tradition that goes back to the work of Arthur Kleinman, a psychiatrist and anthropologist, who revealed the lives of ordinary Chinese through the lens of their illnesses. Such stories unveiled many meanings, not only about the cultural and personal significance of illness itself but also about people's social relationships and the structures of their "social world" (1988, 9).

Health practices, from biomedical, technologically infused activities to alternative care, also run throughout the course of the book. These practices are part of a distinct health culture that has evolved in the San Francisco Bay Area, combining countercultural experiments with immigrant medical pluralism. The people born directly after World War II who came of age during the 1960s and 1970s were seminal in shaping the distinctive health culture, a "competitive edge," for Silicon Valley. Their story sets the stage for the next wave of adults who colonized it, who are now in their mid-thirties and forties. The young people of Silicon Valley, under twenty-five, grew up in this health and work culture, and have internalized its precepts. Productivity, work practices, and the moral values that accompany this distinctive health culture resonate with residents of all ages. Many of the accounts told here reveal how people find ways to thrive in this milieu. The infrastructure of health care also places obstacles that bar some people—the poor, the uninsured, the elderly—from successfully navigating the system. Their stories should also be told.

Having defined embodiment as the defining concept of this ethnography, we will explore what that means. Particular themes run through all the chapters:

- How does distinctive work and health culture of the *place*, Silicon Valley, alter life for this particular group of people?
- How is a culture of *experimentation* realized in each cohort?
- How is *medical pluralism*, derived from the deep diversity and complexity of cultural interactions in this region, made manifest?
- How does the *restaging* of work, family, and health influence life in a particular age group?
- How does the *burden of empowerment*—augmented by an *ethos* of productivity—change the practices of care?

In this chapter, "Embodying Place," we have established changes in work and health that have taken place in the United States, California, and the Silicon Valley region. Since ethnographers rarely encounter generic people, but instead individuals who live in specific times and places, we have to think about the particular qualities of Silicon Valley in the early years of the twenty-first century. Silicon Valley is firmly entrenched in the larger social setting of Northern California, nesting ground to social movements of human transformation. How does that particular piece of cultural heritage change what people do with themselves? The particular attachment to engineering, problem-solving approaches, and affection for technology alters the practices and metaphors of work and health, reinforcing a countercultural tendency toward experimentation. The deep diversity of the region and the global flows of people and ideas restructure how people embody work and tinker with themselves. In this place, the bodies reveal how people "feel capitalism" in the twenty-first century (Wilson and Lande 2005).

The cohort born after World War II is a transitional group that includes those forty-five to sixty-five years old. The leading edge is moving into retirement and the trailing edge is entering late middle age. In Silicon Valley's professional work, these people are highly experienced, and in many ways established the ground rules of the work culture, but less expensive, younger workers are waiting in the wings. That age group also has stressful family and household obligations, to both parents and children. These years constitute the age when it becomes evident that there are "Wearable Parts," the subject of chapter two. Problems with eyes, knees, backs, and skin inten-sify. Obesity, Type-2 diabetes, **coronary artery disease** (CAD), and autoim-mune diseases appear. Fatigue, the enemy of productivity, becomes harder to manage. This is the age of management, across a number of arenas. The *work self* has been created, but must be remolded to fit the changing cir-cumstances. Risk and relationships are managed. Retirements, departures, and deaths begin to take a toll on their social networks.

Children of countercultural revolutions, this cohort was the **first wave** to embrace the combination of biomedical and alternative medicine on a large scale, although they did not begin to do so until they were nearly adults. Their tools for health management include technologies, food, pharmaceuticals, cross-cultural *materia medica*, and spirituality. Chinese medicine, as it is practiced in California, is a critical resource.

The modernist schema of modularity, breaking the world into inter-changeable modules, is used to manage both work and health practices. Modularity is widely practiced, especially by the older cohorts. This leads to further experimentation to buffer the consequences of aging and recap-ture the energy necessary to continue productivity or to find alternatives. Households, material culture, and relationships may all be part of that experimentation. This pattern of management sets up expectations for a high degree of control.

At the same time, people are experimenting with their own life stages. Late onset parenting is not unusual, and this cohort may find themselves approaching retirement while parenting elementary school children. Aging well is the new goal, mitigating the decay of the wearable parts through life-style changes. **Cosmetic surgery** may also subvert age categories. Chronic disease may appear, and it too must be managed.

Chapter three, "In Production," centers on the core workforce in Sili-con Valley. This age group, from twenty-five to forty-five, consists of adults who are establishing professional careers and households. Their work lives have been molded by changes in the global economy in the past generation, particularly intensification, individuation, integration with technology, and global distribution of work. More of the work of the region is devoted to the high-end innovation and service as the manufacturing functions have been relocated. Company policies, practices, and narratives shape the experiences of these workers. The rhythms of their work life are not those of their parents. Work constrains and facilitates their perceptions and management strategies toward time, risk, space, and material culture. It also constrains and facilitates social attitudes toward race, gender, age, and identity. Yet, members of this cohort have grown up with a more intense environment of cultural interaction and borrowing; they are at home with medical diversity. They are the **second wave** of Silicon Valley workers that have become accustomed to deep diversity and persistent experimentation.

In chapter four, "Gearing Up," we see the children who have learned work and health patterns within their own families as U.S. households have become sites of productivity and care again. These youth are native to the conditions of the new economy and constitute the **third wave** of change. Young people, newly on their own, make the transition to self-care and self-direction. Various institutions and ego-centered networks buffer the impact of that transition to some extent. Behaviors and skills learned include gaming and experimentation, building, pruning and maintaining networks, managing their own sexuality, and reconciling competing forms of work morality. These technologically saturated young people are part of an experience economy in which they make themselves interesting, and hence competitive, both formally in a global knowledge economy and in an informal economy of networked reciprocity.

One of the key characteristics of this group is immersion in deep diversity, and a more facile and experimental use of general **cultural competencies** than is seen in their elders. In the San Francisco Bay Area this has meant experimentation with cultural identities as a broader range of cultural behaviors are learned and shuffled. This cultural malleability is part of the crafting of self. Health concepts and modalities of care are also in transition. Parents and peers contribute theories of nutrition, **nutraceuticals**, pharmaceuticals, complementary and alternative medicines. Young people experiment with mitigating, managing, and inviting risk. In addition to self-care, designed to mitigate the lack or lessening of health insurance and access to established medicine, young people can also experiment with bodily augmentation and modification. This age group also experiments with body-centered explanatory systems. Social theories about race, gender, and genetic propensities for disease illustrate how these young people are negotiating and attempting to tinker with their own constraints. How to "beat genetics" is a theme seen in young people who are at risk. Unintended consequences emerge as young people create guerrilla work practices and combine them with new variations of healthy and dangerous lifestyles. Much as the cohort born around World War II have extended lifestyle experiments into their middle years, these young people are establishing a pattern of information inquiry, social validation, and culturally broad experimentation that may change future norms.

Chapter five, "Structural Failure," profiles those people who cannot easily shoulder the burden of empowerment. As aging and chronic conditions ensue, successful navigation of the health care system becomes difficult. The high throughput lifestyle of extraordinary productivity, continuous consumption, and intense activity cannot easily be maintained after retirement. New strategies must emerge. The lessons of the work world are applied to maintaining the body, as people work to survive. While the new patterns of retirement do not necessitate inactivity, people in the postretirement age group face different challenges. After setting up patterns of work activity and lifestyle intensification, the physical impact of aging cannot be denied so easily. CAD, cancer, diabetes, and autoimmune chronic conditions take center stage. Work-based skills in organizing information, constructing practices, and mobilizing networks are harnessed in their final project, staying alive.

The transition to retirement brings an unfamiliar set of bureaucratic constraints as employer-based insurance is displaced by new third-party payers such as Medicare and supplemental insurance. Financial insecurity in this high-cost-of-living area exacerbates the constraints. This is an age where wealth and health are most intimately intertwined. The ability to live with new technologies and prosthetics, to be able to afford fresh food and a comfortable environment separate the elite who can work comfortably on their own longevity from the less affluent, whose experiences are decidedly different. Contrasts between those with and without resources will be made in this section. The oldest members of this cohort have been given an assortment of public and private tools that can be used to prolong and enhance life. However, it cannot be assumed that those following behind them will have access to the same tools. Instead, they will need to rely on their social relationships to buffer the expected loss of infrastructure. — *health?*

Finally, in the last chapter, "Tinkering with the Future," we revisit the notion that new forms of work organization, practice, and morality have placed a premium on productivity, and consider the implications for anthropological approaches to the embodied worker. In this final chapter we will explore Silicon Valley's three natural experiments in linking the body to the work practices of the new economy. The first is derived from the fact that whole bodies, not abstract clusters of skills, are the entities being employed. People are increasingly responsible for integrating all embodied practices—as family members, workers, and well-beings. Second, the structural linkage between employer and health care is being rethought, and job-based insurance care is a phenomenon under siege. Prototypes for **employee-centered wellness programs** are being introduced. Third, deep medical diversity is taking root, combining alternative countercultural care with a wealth of immigrant-based medical beliefs and practices.

Knowledge workers are on the cutting edge of these changes. Silicon Valley, as a mature center for innovation and knowledge work, illustrates how the focus on productivity reorients how people think about their bodies, relationships, their own identities, and the world around them. The San Francisco Bay Area's historical particulars have drawn on the diverse material and conceptual culture of the planet, including *materia medica*. Silicon Valley experiments with technological intensification and augmentation, and increasingly turns from concrete institutions to decentralized, networked organizations to manage life's dilemmas. Implications abound for employers, families, educators and especially the ever-expanding players in health economy. Employers may drive the need for productivity, but they also provide sites for the mitigation of the unintended consequences.

The reformulation of the employer-employee relationship vis-à-vis health penetrates workers' lives as never before. While this may prove effective in shaping health outcomes, it brings the purview of the workplace into the most intimate details of personal life. Self-monitoring is coupled with the ubiquitous gaze of technology-based employer surveillance. What you eat, where you park, how many steps you took today, and how you feel become legitimate areas of inquiry in employee-centric health care strategies. Companies, as new sites of health care, are already proliferating in the health marketplace. Company wellness programs "reduce illness and injuries, not only for the employees but also for their families" (Mitchell 2004, 38). Tracking such issues as family leave claims, lost productivity time due to particular impairments, work groups and work shifts with the highest lost time and medical costs is critical to mapping problems and creating managerial policy (ibid., 36). How do individuals negotiate these pressures? How will corporations? Workers use their workplaces to get access to resources and intelligence about health. Family and friends are fundamentally a part of the building of self. Ironically, the vulnerability of individuation both intensifies individuality and ties individuals more intimately to kith and kin for support.

Each of the critical themes of the book—distinctiveness of place, experimentation, medical pluralism, life restaging, and individuation—manifests itself differently in each age group. The first wave, the people born immediately after World War II, laid the foundation for change among those who followed them. The changes in work practice, intercultural interaction, and the very conceptualization of health made it possible for their children to create a new framework for working, being, and well-being.

[handwritten notes at top of page:]

- taking values of work re Memocuatory + innovation into health practice + back
- body as wearable
- She is member of the first wave (post WW2) 1946-84
  ↳ created (with the cohort preceding) the knowledge econ.
- neolinguistic programming = affirmations
- aging has element of choice ←
  ↳ metaphors of nature + manufacture ⟶
- sandwich gen
- cradle to grave = planned obsolesence

2   Wearable Parts

Fifty years old.
I still spend my time
Screwing nuts down on bolts.
At the shadow pool,
Children are sleeping,
And a lover I've lived with for years,
True night.
One cannot stay too long awake
In this dark

—Snyder 1983, "True Night," 45

Margaret Ginsberg, Embodying the First Wave

Margaret Ginsberg is a San Francisco Bay Area native, born in 1956, and her life exemplifies the countercultural and technological story of the region. Margaret is a technical writer with deep experience in the high-tech industry, daughter of a physicist at one at the region's several national laboratories. She tells of her father's transformation after he took LSD under the care of Timothy Leary. Overnight, her upbringing went from "ultraconservative" to "ultraliberal," her mother telling her to "try everything once." Margaret traveled to India, Thailand, and Nepal with her intended, a soon-to-be high-achieving executive in computing—and a science fiction novelist. Margaret returned to be married on a horse in a redwood grove, her Jewish relatives and his Catholic fisher folk equally aghast. Like many others of her cohort, she had her child late in life, when she was thirty-seven. She expected her life to unfold along a rather predictable timeline, but that is not how it happened. She reflects, "It's so funny, because I see so many people around me just like the situation that I'm in, where they have children late and it changes their life. . . . For me it's like, there are these stages and there's no time line on it." She herself has lived through several life stages already—the college stage, the travel stage, and in building her Silicon Valley career, the money stage. She *would* like to write a novel before she "dies," but for now she works with her husband on his novel. Maybe her dream work will be published, maybe not, but it is on her life's "to do" list. She feels drawn to the past through art and philosophy, and to the future through technology. One of her coworkers remarked on this tension and gave her a toy symbolizing that she is a "wolf in sheep's clothing." She is "a New Age person that's buried under all this disguise of technology."

Margaret is now a technical writer at a major Internet hardware firm, but she has gone through many career incarnations—manager, writer, trainer. She has been in "unhealthy" companies, such as one "funded with venture capital. It runs out of money because it doesn't have proper management or proper products, or it doesn't bring its product to market on time within the window that it needs to go in. Or one that is already failing for whatever reasons and is going down the tubes and it could just as easily shut its doors." The pink slip that delivers the message of impending unemployment is like a critical diagnosis, an indication of poor corporate health. "Quick and dirty" production practices shocked her; she would like to demand better fiscal hygiene. It took her a long time to realize that the poor health of the company did not need to lead to stress and ill health in her own life. Nearby agencies offered training to help her transition to new jobs, and she learned how to look for a "healthy company. What to look for in the kind of people I wanted to work with, what to look for in a job." Margaret uses health metaphors to understand the uncertain new economy. At the same time, she explains that she gets sick from the stress induced by the volatility of the high-technology industry.

She encountered environmental health problems peculiar to working in the high-technology sector. In one company, she encountered pet iguanas that lived in the cubicles. In another, "All these terrible chemicals would pour out, pour all over the floor . . . out to where my office cube was . . . and they would use wet vacuums to vacuum it all up . . . and I would wonder if I should change my shoes. It was just like, really weird stuff." She began to look at her life as if it were a science fiction movie, mentally commenting on the strange activities around her in the early years of Silicon Valley, but staying afloat within it. Detachment was her mental tactic for emotional survival.

When her child was born, she joined a mother's group and has stayed connected to them by email. They go camping together. In her youth, she would go camping. Then, the Sierras were much less polluted, but going now still provides a connection to nature. "I draw my spirituality from this nature." She has a plant in her cubicle to give her oxygen and remind her of the outdoors. American Transcendentalism, rendering nature sublime and spiritual, is alive and well in Margaret. While nature is considered a powerful force, so are words.

When she went to the University of California, Margaret became involved with the neurolinguistic programming movement, as did her husband. A product of charismatic academics at Berkeley and Santa Cruz, including the anthropologist Gregory Bateson, neurolinguistic programming became a critical piece of the self-help movement, drawing attention to the power of language and mental models. Margaret became sensitive to how people frame themselves in language and thought. For example, calling a damaged heart "bad," reframes a neutral descriptive disease state into a moral failing. For optimal mental health, such framing is to be avoided. The process itself can be generalized, as it was by self-help personality Anthony Robbins, into management and seminars for "success."

Margaret works on her physical body as well. Drawing on a deep background of massage and dance, Margaret looks at her own forty-something body, and then encourages her high-technology colleagues to work out with her. This combination of alternative lifestyle and technological immersion lays the groundwork for meshing herbal tea and biomedicine, and playfully and consciously experimenting with cognition while searching for efficient solutions.

Margaret's quest for aging well is a story we see throughout her cohort. She harnesses the tools developed in her youth that fold countercultural beliefs and practices and technoscientific experimentation. Her agemates, and their immediate elders, developed the companies and practices that defined the new economy in which the notions of meritocracy and innovation are valued—even if the practice of these sentiments falls short. They readily transpose metaphors from these new work practices to health, and back again, in which individual action is celebrated.

They are also aging into a heightened awareness of their own bodily vulnerabilities. Although she is in the second wave cohort, Veeda Ferrazzi succinctly summarizes the dilemma as she imagines herself getting older. Veeda comments that all her body parts are not aging at the same rate. Some parts are still supple and strong, others hurt after gardening or a long day at the computer. Back, knees, teeth, eyes—all are vulnerable to the ravages of time. Veeda reflects, "My God! We just take these eyes and teeth and things for granted! . . . Yeah, these are wearable parts."

Not Quite the Revolution

Margaret's cohort was born after World War II, in the period between 1946 and 1964; people in this age set lived through collective changes that transformed the American experience. Access to higher education, control over family planning, and the demands of work changed as they reached adulthood (Moen and Roehling 2005, 137; Vian 2007). One of the difficulties people in Margaret's cohort face in navigating their moral landscape is that they themselves were instrumental in changing the rules that had prevailed during their youth. They are drawing on distinct frames—metaphors that structure our thoughts and feelings—of morality and knowledge that help them construct their decisions. These frameworks, or foundational schema, include notions of goodness. Some of these frames were strongly in place in the households in which they were reared. Others were innovative constructs, often derived from historic movements, such as nineteenth-century Transcendentalism, that were given new life and meaning in the sixties. Self-sacrifice is good, especially for women. Self-discipline—mastering appetites and physical practices—is virtuous.

However, the region's decades-long Dionysian experimentation in foods, sensualism, sexuality, and cognitive experiences challenged old frameworks of virtue. Sex, drugs, and rock and roll revolutionized the sense of self that was culturally allowable. New immigrants brought new foods and health practices in the late 1960s, and the sojourns of people in this cohort into the wider world broadened their culinary, medical, and philosophical horizons. The revival of "natural" healing in the seventies created a "countercuisine" that was meant to help consumers survive an apocalypse, cure disease, offer sensual delight, and create an atmosphere of playful fun. Ethnic and regional cooking was revitalized (Belasco 2007, 4). Although this first wave of cultural revolutionaries helped start these changes, they were not fully socialized into that alternative experience; they came to it as adolescents or adults.

I myself am a member of this cohort, born in 1953. I did not realize that it was possible to eat vegetables that were not cooked into an amorphous mass until I was exposed to "steamed" vegetables and nutty brown rice as an adult. A childhood klutz in secondary school competitive sports, I learned that dance, yoga, and *taiji* were well within my capability as a grown woman, and that there is considerable pleasure in attempting embodied disciplines. This first wave is not native to these new cultural frames, and they sometimes find themselves navigating very different forms of knowl-edge—from scientific inquiry to intuitive inspiration.

There are, depending on how they are counted, approximately 77 million members of Margaret's cohort in the United States. This group routinely got measles, chicken pox, mumps, and other infectious diseases as children, and grew up with John F. Kennedy's physical fitness movement in their elementary and secondary schools. Before this lot came of age in the 1960s and 1970s, American tertiary education was for the elite. They were the first generation to go to college en masse (Kirsch and Jeffery 2003, 2, 10–11). Constrained by military draft policies in the Vietnam War, men found majoring in engineering or anthropology preferable to serving in Southeast Asia. Young women, particularly those born in the late fifties, found themselves in universities at the dawn of the women's movement. International travel was affordable as never before, and, as for Margaret, traveling to distant cultures was a common *rite de passage* between education and career for this cohort's youth.

Between 1980 and 1995, the birthrate for women in their early forties increased 81 percent (ibid., 10). With easier access to birth control and advanced education, parenthood could come early, late, or not at all. The children act as social bridges between parents of different age cohorts. Connecting to the parents of your children's friends could mean relating to people your own age, or reaching across cohorts to much younger parents.

The people born after World War II are aging into more complex caretaking roles. The home, rather than hospitals or other institutions, has once again become a site for caretaking. Late children and long-lived parents mean increased caregiving by this age cohort. Approximately 14 million Americans are now caring for an elderly relative. Those caretakers are either elderly themselves or members of this age group (Bookman 2004, 149–50). The person they are caring for may be across the street or a major flight away. In any case, the caretakers' work is disrupted by the need to manage an extra load of medical visits.

It is most useful to think of this first wave's experience as a cross-fertilization of cohort effect, experiencing broadly similar events in cultural history, and the aging process itself. When thinking about this group as a worker segment, this is crucial. This cohort, with their elders, cocreated the knowledge economy in the seventies—a new kind of work. In Silicon Valley that work centered on technical creativity, but new niches grew to service that sector. Margaret is not the archetypical Silicon Valley engineer, but she and her husband participate in a larger work culture that values precision, creativity, and management. Their day-to-day experiences as knowledge workers are based on the flexible and intensive work practices born in the Silicon Valley high-tech environment. The world of work was being remade during the very years when they learned to be workers. Yet, they grew up expecting one sort of work—predictable and orderly—which disappeared on them midcareer. For that reason, over time this cohort has grown to view work more pragmatically and with less idealism. As they age, this first wave increasingly wants to find worth outside of work (Smola and Sutton 2002, 379). They also have a broader range of responsibilities outside the home.

The expected work staging also changed for this first wave. The "lock-step" system—(1) prepare-for-work, (2) be paid for work, and (3) retire—is breaking down. Members of this cohort are likely not only to be caring for children and parents but also to be working into their advanced years while trying to care for them! Just as this cohort approach retirement, that life stage becomes ever more problematic. Labor force participation for people over fifty-five, particularly women, is increasing. More educated workers, those who need income, and those who require work-based health benefits postpone retirement, or change the way in which they work (Copeland 2007, 1–2). The emerging cultural ideal for successful aging requires engagement in ongoing activity—new jobs, new patterns of part-time work, and meaningful community work (Moen and Roehling 2005, 130–54).

Members of this cohort are now aging, and their **chronic disease burden** is mounting. Heart disease, metabolic diseases, and cancer are increasingly common experiences for them. As they grow older, the median age of people with Type 2 diabetes is creeping downward to embrace their generation (Schoenberg et al. 2005, 172). New chronic diseases of perplexing **etiology**—such as chronic fatigue, fibromyalgia, and **multiple chemical sensitivity** (MCS)—complicate the lives of this aging cohort and confound their care (Thompson and Troester 2002, 557; Lipson 2004). As they reach sixty-five, they have fewer disabilities than did the generation before them, but they still feel the ravages of time (Vian 2007, 1). Hearing, eyesight, and knee problems are here to stay for those born in 1964 or before. The wearability of body parts is coming home to roost.

Many of the features of this first wave of revolutionaries can be found throughout the United States, most broadly in American urban environments. The San Francisco Bay Area was seminal in this transformation in the 1960s and 1970s. Stanford's technological optimists and LSD advocates, the Merry Pranksters—Ken Kesey, Jerry Garcia from the Grateful Dead, Stewart Brand of the *Whole Earth Catalog* and *CoEvolution Quarterly,* along with many others—fused countercultural attitude, experimentation, and creation. Organizations such as the Augmentation Research Center (ARC), the Stanford Research Institute (SRI), the Palo Alto Research Center (PARC), and the Homebrew Computing Club juxtaposed technological innovation with countercultural play (Turner 2006, 64, 106). Outside of the not-yet-named Silicon Valley, Berkeley and San Francisco were centers for the natural food movement, integrating what could arguably be called protoecological movement beliefs.

Natural was good. Of course, "nature" is a slippery term that at times refers to ingredients, at other times to ecological attitudes, while simultaneously referring vaguely and nostalgically to preindustrial practices (Belasco 2007, 41). "Plastic" processed food is unhealthful and morally unclean. White foods, from Wonder Bread to Cool Whip, were emblematic of white politics and the whitewashing of America's woes. Gary Snyder, the iconic Beat poet, defended the rights of trees in People's Park in Berkeley, helping to transform the meaning of the word "ecology" from a subfield in biology to a political position (ibid., 21–24, 28).

San Francisco led the way to a new cuisine that borrowed from inexpensive ethnic food, natural ingredients, and cultivated aesthetics to create California's fusion cuisine. The food was to be fun to prepare and yet demanding a certain skill and threshold of refinement. This cuisine was connected to California's class and ethnic politics. It gentrified ethnic food and made eating peasant cuisine nostalgic. Organic food, grown without pesticides, was not only cleaner but also politically superior because it was not poisoning farm workers. As in China, "[A]ll food is so political" (Farquhar 2002, 79–81). Californian cuisine is increasingly linked with considerations of ecological impact. The Bay Area could afford to promote localized food because of the abundant agricultural bounty in the Coastal and Central valleys. From Napa's wines to Monterey's strawberries, fresh flavors were available for experimentation. This *cuisine nouvelle* was also therapeutic; meals become medicinal. Eating replenishes life force, whether that is thought of as Ayurvedic *prana* or East Asian *qi*. Processed food is devoid of this vitality. A beautiful salad, artfully arranged, feeds both body and soul. A sip of locally brewed dark beer nourishes the spirit as well as the senses.

Members of this first wave of change, especially those in the San Francisco Bay Area, are broadly associated with a host of health-related revolutions. Born in the late forties and fifties, this cohort is associated with the alternative food movements. The median birth year for organic food consumers is 1957 (Kirsch and Jeffery 2003, 50). Coupled with the post-1965 immigration influx of people and their foods, and the widespread travel abroad, the cohort's smorgasbord, particularly in places like the San Francisco Bay Area, draws from a global cornucopia of choices (see Vian 2007, 1). This is the generation that shepherded in a food revolution, transform-

ing the habits of a small but long-standing American health food movement into a major economic market.

The changes of the first wave include being open to cultural experimentation. Much of this experimentation is countercultural, but it also reflects
people playing with adapting cultural practices that are made more available through immigration and globalization. The presence of many diverse
medical traditions intersects with the countercultural adoption of ancient
healing practices. The members of this cohort are also restaging their own
life courses as they move through changing family and work roles.

The onus of "empowerment" for individual productivity fell to this
cohort in the middle of their careers. They began their working and family
roles supported by a variety of institutional structures, only to see them
lose credibility. In their youth, they could imagine bonds of mutual loyalty
between themselves and their employers. This tacit, and largely imaginary,
social contract faded as they hit middle age. This first wave both shaped
and adapted to these larger political and economic changes.

*relationship between bio Medical + well being care ie
food + Mental State*

Ron Little, Open to Experimenting

The members of this first wave of change show a propensity for experimentation and questioning traditional American categories of self-management and identity. We will closely reexamine the local experience of
diversity, as it influences the range of options this first wave view as viable
alternatives in caring for others and themselves. Given the deep diversity of
the region, and the rich history of alternative experimentation in the larger
Bay Area, health care choices transcend the usual descriptions of medical
pluralism. Members of this educated cohort—a descriptor appropriate for
those who have been attracted to work in Silicon Valley—want to *age well*.
Aging well may mean overturning the cultural assumptions of people born
before World War II. Is sixty old, or middle-aged? Aging well may be complicated by the need to care for others: ill children, spouses that are not
aging as well, and parents. We will extend our inquiry more deeply into the
modes of experimentation around food and other forms of health.

Ron Little is in his fifties now, but he is the father of two small children, ages six and eight. He is a marine biologist who works in a regulatory agency that manages wetlands. His work schedule is fairly predictable; he works nine long days and gets a Friday off every two weeks, punctuated by field trips to San Francisco's Bay—either literally on the bay itself, or at a nearby landfill. The experimental method is not only a part of his professional work; it is integral to his life. He enjoys his walk to the Caltrain station to commute. He tries out different alternatives; his daily exercise is important to him. Ron has already had heart bypass surgery, and he must improve his lung function with gentle exercise, healthful diet, and regular medication.

Ron grew up on meat and potatoes and hated vegetables. "Vegetables—get them out of here! Fruit—get it out of here! Give me a hamburger, cheeseburger, French fries and a milkshake and that's fine. Or Cheerios." He had asthma when he was a child. He was hooked on his inhaler and needed to get weekly allergy shots. Then, at twelve, he decided it was psychosomatic and "did a self-experiment and I proved myself right, that it was not all psychosomatic, but most of it was." He played sports in high school and was active during the summer. After graduating from high school he went to Sweden and "discovered food is good!" The rite of passage for his cohort, international travel, opened up new avenues of culinary experimentation.

Ron's "health awakening" occurred after he moved to Australia. There his mentor, Mick, introduced him to Eastern philosophy, yoga, acupuncture, and Zen practice. Psychologist Richard Alpert—later known as Ram Dass—who had been part of Timothy Leary's and Ken Kesey's intellectual cadre—remains an influence in Ron's life. While still a meat and potatoes man at heart, in Australia Ron learned to eat new foods, such as brown rice. Ron laughs remembering that he thought, "What the heck is brown rice?" He ate vegetables because they were more affordable than meat. He was in the water exercising every day. Mick also got Ron to run on a regular basis. Ron began to learn that managing "your mental state" is integral to health. While these were important discoveries to be resurrected in his middle age, his health practices were those of a young man. At that time he didn't think about his cholesterol, because "when you're in your early twenties you're invincible, so what difference does it make?"

After Ron left Australia in the eighties he attended the self-transformation **est** seminars of Werner Erhard. Like Margaret's neurolinguistic programming, these seminars presented cognitive tools, "technologies of transformation," that highlighted the relationship of choice and responsibility as the frameworks by which individuals understand their actions. Two-weekend workshops—sixty hours of EST training—"made me very aware of the fact that I am responsible for everything I do. I have to accept everything I do because I choose everything. And that really sank in—that I choose what I do. You're responsible for your own actions. And I pretty much live by that." Years later, this frames how he thinks about his coronary artery disease management. He had made choices; they had consequences. Ron can make new choices with new outcomes.

When he first had chest pains, the physicians attributed it to his asthma. Luckily, his wife, Kate, had a different medical insurance plan that also covered him, and he got a second opinion from a cardiologist. In 1996 he "went under the knife and got it fixed." Of course, the surgery was not the end of the story, but the event that triggered new choices. Ron takes a string of medications, niacin, baby aspirin, Lovastatin, Zestril, and Diltia; he reads food labels and chooses foods that have low levels of cholesterol, fat, and sodium. "Much more fish comes into this house. A lot more fruits and vegetables come into this house than before." At work, he will go to lunch at Baja Fresh to get fish or Noah's Bagels—substituting hummus for cream cheese.

The relationship between his food and pharmaceutical choices is complex. He wants to wean himself from pills. "I don't want to be a walking pharmacy. I see old people that have this bag of pills all over the place, and I just don't want to do that. But I've come to realize that if I want to live anywhere near what I would consider a normal life, then I must be willing to supplement to some degree." He doesn't want to change his diet radically, because he likes "different flavors," and to eliminate them would be boring, making it that much harder to adhere to a healthful lifestyle. So he takes his pills and still eats his Mexican food, but leaves off the cheese. Fish tacos are enough for him. As a parent he knows that his "kids eat junk," and if the household diet is more healthful, then everyone will benefit. "But we try not to overdo it." He monitors himself so that if the need to change is apparent, he will make his regime stricter. He balances convenience and the need for behavioral change, using the alchemy of pharmaceuticals.

His workplace supports his self-care regime; they have an on-site wellness center where he does stretches and abdominal crunches and tones his body with weights. If he were so inclined, they would pay for part of his membership at a health club, but he prefers the convenience of the workplace gym. His aerobic activities—walking, biking, jogging—he prefers to do outside, although his knees do bother him. At the moment, exercising on the weekends is a problem, since that is when his children's activities are scheduled. The morality of making family time competes with the imperative for exercise.

Ron also works on his inner "spiritual" and cognitive state, drawing on his experiences with self-actualization. Ron comments, "I think it's very important for your health to be in a positive frame of mind—better energy inside, better karma. . . . It just gets you in a bad place all the time to see the negative side of it." Using this approach, notice how Ron talks about his heart: "My heart's fine. Just bad plumbing is what it is. . . . Take it for what it's worth and move on." The words themselves have power. A "bad heart" is a judgment, "bad plumbing" is a neutral description of a technical problem, and such problems can be corrected.

The management of his disease blends and merges with the management of his life. It is utterly integrated with his role as a husband, father, and worker. It also reflects that particular quality we will seen again and again in the younger cohorts—the affinity for experimentation. Ron is aware of this and attributes it both to his scientific background and his countercultural one: "I'm very open to experimenting. I guess that's the science in me, but I've always been an experimenter. Born out of the sixties, I've been an experimenter!"

Explanatory Frameworks, Hybrid Etiologies

While members of Ron's and Margaret's cohort did not discover the Eastward-looking transcendental philosophies associated with alternative healing, they certainly resurrected them and integrated them into their parenting, consumption, and self-care practices. Yoga, *taiji*, and herbal over-the-counter supplements were infused into the practices of this age group, at least once they became adults. They are at the cusp, with one foot in biomedical orthodoxies and the other in organic and alternative experiments.

I have encountered the merging of counterculture and technoculture in my own ethnographic work in California since the 1980s. In studying the holistic healers of Southern California, I would find Euro-American shamans and psychics who had day jobs as Silicon Valley engineers. In the 1990s, when I began to collect the stories of Silicon Valley workers, I again would find that a fascination with technology and a romantic countercultural valorization of nature went hand in hand. Throughout this book we will see examples of people engaging in rational problem-solving, passionately affixed to biomedical details, while simultaneously embracing alternative healing methods.

This first wave, who had lived through these changes, have at their disposal a range of beliefs and practices—different forms of knowledge about managing health and the embodied self—that come from their experiences over the course of the decades. They are not native to the revolutions, but have learned to use other frames of reference. There are at least four competing and complementary **medical epistemologies** of the body on which they can draw.

One form of knowledge is strictly biomedical. The educational level of Silicon Valley is such that many people have—or have access to people who have—a working understanding of physiology and chemistry. They can use a search engine to successfully read and *understand* the many sources of information available from the Internet. There are clear gatekeepers of this form of knowledge, centered on physician expertise.

The second framework draws on a domestic form of public health that has been in place for a century. That set of medical beliefs and practices synthesized the emerging understanding of the role of pathogens and the already existing hygienic movement. This clean-and-germ-free approach was directed to the home and the women who were the familial caretakers (Tomes 1997). Regular meals, scrubbed rooms, fresh air, and clean-living bodies would translate into health in this philosophy. This is domestic knowledge, learned at the mother's knee, but shaped by larger discourses of public health, product marketing, and consumer reaction.

The third medical epistemology available—promoted initially by this cohort—is the deep medical diversity that emerged from immigration, the onset of global travel, and the countercultural embrace of alternative healing. This is the most amorphous and complex of the beliefs. It can draw on "traditional" remedies such as hot honey lemon drinks for coughs, or quasi-biomedical blood work which suggests that acidic blood requires a change in diet toward more vegetables and fruits. The range of therapeutic interventions matches the complexity of the **Naturalistic etiologies** that emphasize balance, self-care, food, and movement. Expertise is diffuse. The fracturing of scientific expert knowledge and trust is evident in the stories of people who embrace this alternative approach (see Hunt 2003, 170). Icons such as Andrew Weil or Deepak Chopra form a visible source of alternative expertise. The underlying rationale for use comes most from the evident success of individual family, friends, and coworkers, experimenting with particular practices.

Finally, and intimately associated with alternative health practices, is an increased consciousness that a person—body, mind, and spirit—will reflect the larger environment. This is an old idea, derived from archaic naturalist medical beliefs that the microcosm is a reflection of the macrocosm, suggesting that "my body will directly reflect the health of my environment." This idea has been given new life and sophistication as our means of measuring the health of the environment improves. Complex biochemical tests are done institutionally and broadcast by biocitizens via the Internet.[1] The Silicon Valley Toxic Tour, on the Silicon Valley Toxic Coalition website maps groundwater contamination and school sites. Consumers make their own assessments of commercial food's purity and share their opinions globally. Safe Food International, affiliated with the Center for Science in the Public Interest, runs a clearinghouse wiki to facilitate the dissemination of such information.

Organic, green, sustainable health is appearing on the epistemological horizon. New sources of information—from computer wielding biocitizens, such as the Silicon Valley Toxics Coalition, to governmental reports—form the foundation for activism. At the individual level consumers make their assessments on green marketing using certified labels, such as the USDA Organic certification. Remember the multiple meanings of "nature" in use in countercultural food. Is "nature" an ingredient, transcendental philosophy, or historical preindustrial practice? Any of these frames of reference might catapult a food into the category "natural." Organic heirloom tomatoes are triply natural: grown without pesticides, from prehybrid ancestral roots, and made into wholesome, aesthetic, spirit-nourishing salads. Moreover, they provide lycopene, a potent nutritional antioxidant!

Beyond the medical constructs that inform healing practice is another offspring of the counterculture—the hedonistic embrace of pleasure, desire, and sensuality. Part of this ecstatic philosophy is the pursuit of happiness, not as contentment but as bliss. Eat chocolate, for it contains theobromine, which is a vasodilator and antioxidant. Select brands that are shade-grown, organic, and practice fair trade, so that it is ecologically and socially justifiable. However, the chocolate must be aromatic, flavorful, distinctive, and induce near-ecstasy. Artisan chocolate is more than a healthful food; it draws on a form of knowledge known as *taste*, a culturally constructed and sensual practice that sets the standards for the smorgasbord from which this cohort, and their children, select their options.

The San Francisco Bay Area has been a magnet for East Asian immigration since the mid-nineteenth-century Gold Rush. The Chinese name for San Francisco—*Jin Shan* (Gold Mountain)—reflects the historicity of the connection. However, the 1965 changes to immigration policy had a profound impact on the region, bringing in new populations of ethnic Chinese Vietnamese refugees and Taiwanese-educated engineers and students from the People's Republic who stayed to build Silicon Valley. With these moving bodies came diverse ideas of illness, wellness, and healing.

One of the medical practices imported, along with the immigrants and sojourners, is **qigong**. Often superficially called Chinese yoga, *qigong* is a set of breathing and cognitive exercises, postures, and movements designed to work with the energy centers of the body and harness the flow of *qi* throughout the **meridians** that are also used in acupuncture. Feeling *qi* is to feel the life that flows inside and all around us. *Qigong* is intimately connected with martial arts, especially in inner forms such as *taiji*, as well as the practice of traditional Chinese medicine (TCM). *Qigong* and *taiji* practices work the body, but also sensitize the practitioner of these arts to feel energy as a tangible living force. It is a rejuvenating practice used in China the way Americans use coffee (Chen 2003, 47). *Qigong's* popularity in China grew during the post-Maoist reforms as a form of self-help that lent itself to the market economy, and to rebuilding the "traditional" Chinese culture that had been damaged during the worst ravages of the Cultural Revolution.

The Enduring Pine Healing Center, Institutionalizing Deep Medical Diversity

[handwritten margin note: — view of alternative medicine practitioners → traditional medicine as qualitative]

In the early nineties, one of the three top practitioners of medical *qigong*, Dr. Zheng, visited the United States, lecturing largely to Chinese immigrants, their children, and grandchildren. He gave long lectures describing *qi*, drawing on both physics and traditional medicine to frame his talk. His demonstration of *qi* in the crowd in San Francisco "was electric, with members erupting with sudden cries and swaying back and forth in their seats. Some shone with ecstatic smiles of delight, others shook with deep, heavy sobs" (ibid., 165–66). Zheng connected to *qigong* adherents of Chinese ancestry and those who practice alternative medicine without being born to the culture.

Among Zheng's students is Jerry Allen Johnson, a teacher-practitioner in Pacific Grove, near Monterey, who runs a *qigong* school and Daoist temple (Johnson 2008). He is a culture broker who translates his training in China for his American practitioners. His students practice in the Silicon Valley. The Enduring Pine Healing Center, named for a symbol of longevity and Daoist philosophy, is one of the centers of medical *qigong* practice in Silicon Valley.[2] Founded by Charles Sheridan, a local man in his late thirties, the center is a site for medical *qigong* practice, Chinese face reading, Chinese philosophy, nutrition, yoga, and, of course, *taiji*. Charles found the path to healing *qi* through the martial arts. Charles has Chinese and non-Chinese clients in his center. While all express respect, Charles and his fellow practitioner, Celia Batista, find they have to make a special effort to demonstrate their knowledge to the Chinese students—their cultural authority does not come automatically. Charles learns it is easier to impress the non-Chinese students with his martial arts credentials and knowledge of traditional Chinese medical practices (such as tongue, smell, and facial feature diagnosis). Such practices require that he educate his clientele about the logic and application of Chinese healing.

Celia, also in her mid-thirties, is a petite, blonde Puerto Rican Latina who grew up in the Southeast and moved to California to get more education in Daoism and create a practice. Celia came to medical *qigong* through her own health practices. She began with *taiji* and then explored natural healing as she "trained for delivery" during her pregnancy. She even competed in *taiji* tournaments when she was eight months pregnant. She realized that, with training, she could reach out to help other people, beyond her own family. So she became a Chinese medical *qigong* practitioner. She finds that she needs to "defend" her right to wear Chinese style clothes and practice Chinese medicine without being and speaking Chinese (see Lau 2000, 120). She felt especially marginalized when she visited China. She has few Asian clients, except those who are generations away from arrival. Celia reflects that "for *qigong* class or a *taiji* class, you have to be really good. Otherwise, they won't learn from you, they won't go to you." On the other hand, while some clients would reject anything Chinese, most are open to the experience. Celia comments on the assets and drawbacks of her Bay Area clientele, and inadvertently describes its deep medical diversity:

> I think one of the things that strikes me is that California is really open to alternative healing and different modalities, which is beautiful. There is such a huge movement of people who are open to it. . . . "Yeah, I'll go for my weekly massage and I love taking care of myself, being organic." That is definitely California. . . . So I do appreciate that quality in Californians. . . . As far as practicing . . . I wish that people would really take a little more time to go deeper with what's available and what they can be offered, because there are really some incredible people here.

Many are willing to embrace Chinese theory as an alternative model to biomedicine. Others balk at too much authenticity and shy away from "exotic" therapies. For the former, she might go in depth explaining and using fire cups to stimulate or sedate acupuncture points (see Photograph 2). She would explain the underlying logic of the dominant problem she sees—deficiency of kidney fire, the loss of adrenal function, brought on by the continual battle against exhaustion. Celia says that kidney fire deficiency is the problem for "ninety percent of the people who walk in through this door. They are malnourished, dehydrated, lack rest, and are overworked." She explores the metaphysical side of Daoism only for her most adept clients. Celia sensitizes them to the ethereal harmful entities that can be drawn to people who abuse themselves; she gives her clients herbal concoctions, behavioral education, and mental-spiritual tools for self-defense. Alternative medicine's long flirtation with transcendental metaphysics and spiritualism opens this door. Some of her clients are less open to TCM; for them she might simply use suction cups and massage and emphasize stress reduction and relaxation—common popular biomedical concepts.

Yet the clients, who place medical *qigong* next to a host of other practices in their repertoire, rarely go deeply into any one system. Celia knows that the medical *qigong* community in the San Francisco Bay Area is diverse and complex. Most clients are not aware of the expertise available in the region, nor are they conscious of the intense competition between practitioners. Nonetheless, her clients can walk in public spaces throughout the region at dawn and see Chinese immigrant elders doing *taiji*. Shopping malls in east San Jose, Cupertino, and Milpitas have traditional Chinese herbal stores. Even the Latino *botánicas* carry Chinese herbal products. Chinese immigrants are comforted by the pervasive atmosphere of "Sino-California." Thus Chineseness is normalized for other kinds of Californians and to be taken for granted. This dynamic is the epitome of deep medical diversity.

Sofia, at the leading edge of the first wave cohort, is sixty years old and just beginning to become a medical *qigong* practitioner. She is an engineer and scientist by training, with degrees in physics and electrical engineering. Sofia's long history of personal experimentation brought her to the Enduring Pine Healing Center, where she is an intern. She was initially interested in meditation and did not see *taiji* and *qigong* as healing arts. She saw the connection to health as she reduced her "stress" and has "gotten more relaxed." When she first took a class on medical *qigong* she was skeptical; she did not understand the metaphysical aspects. Sophia says, "I am really very open to alternative therapies because I used a lot of alternative therapies. . . . But . . . I wasn't used to this kind." Then she realized that the underlying logic of *qigong* was the same as that of acupuncture, which she did understand. She started to see people respond to it. Enthusiastically she recounts:

> That guy came in last week. He can hardly walk. . . . He couldn't see he had such a bad headache. His eyes were all bloodshot. He couldn't focus. He was in pain. He left one hour later. He could walk. His eyes could focus. He was pain free. Poor guy. No medical insurance. He's lost everything because exhausted all his resources. He's lost his home. He's lost his wife, both his parents. They lost their business. They were burglarized. His parents folded up from the stress. Where's he got to go? He's here.

The value of alternative practice to those marginalized by biomedicine is important to Sofia. After she retired from her engineering career, she toyed with landscaping as a second career, "but it doesn't give anything back. I'm sixty years old. I want to be doing something that gives back a little . . . within the circle of influence that I have, that I can make a difference. Because if every person made a difference within [his or her] circle of influence, it would change the world." She works for immigrant rights at a day labor center, having encountered immigrants in her landscaping work. Sofia recalls that she grew up with a vision that she should have an impact on the world. She has come to see that having an impact within her own small sphere of influence will help her become healthier as well as establish social justice. Having been an engineer and a landscaper, Sofia says that her "third career" in alternative healing is "really changing my life." Sofia, like others in her cohort, longs to change the world, or at least, herself.

The practices at Enduring Pine highlight the challenges of intertwining biomedical and medically plural healing systems. Some of the assumptions in spiritual healing are inherently incompatible with the biomedical approach, which validates only physical reality. A radical embrace of the natural, perceived as "spiritually pure," would incline adherents to refuse the use of monoclonal antibodies or radical prostheses. On the other hand, advocates of biomedicine and household hygiene would find *shivambu kalpa*, the Ayurvedic practice of drinking urine to recycle nutrients, utterly disgusting. Nonetheless, there is substantial overlap between the medical systems in terms of acceptable daily practices. Whether approaching health from a spiritual, public health, or biomedical perspective, all embrace self-denial or moderation as a fundamental practice. Smoking cigarettes is not good for you in any of these belief systems.

However, to comprehend how this pluralistic experimentation works, we need to understand modular thinking, a curiosity of American cognition. Such frames reflect a structural propensity to break the world into modules or interchangeable chunks of behavior. Such thinking allows people to mix and match from a variety of health traditions. Practicing medical pluralism necessitates considerable translation work. The metrics by which biomedicine measures health, almost certainly **quantitative**, must mesh with more ephemeral **qualitative** metrics of other medical traditions, such as wellness, vitality, and the ability to be creatively productive.

Modularity and Menopause

The cohort of this first wave, raised in the late forties through the early sixties, is observably modern in its cognitive organization. Industrial life, particularly in the United States, requires a certain kind of mental organization that has been referred to as modularity. Modularity is a broad design principle that reflects and reinforces the everyday reality of Americans, especially during the twentieth century (Blair 1988, 1–5). Jazz is a peculiarly American form of music with interchangeable modules subject to improvisation. An American university education, unlike its Oxbridge British equivalent, consists of interchangeable units, called classes, that build larger modules—majors. Successive degrees build careers. People in those careers regulate their lives in time modules, based on the business quarter. They may drift from religious experience to religious experience, treating their sojourn in a particular church or temple as an interchangeable module (ibid., 116–17). Houses are the modules of neighborhoods, rooms the modules of houses, and furniture the modules for rooms (Shore 1996, 118–19). Pragmatism governs how the modules are used, holding that underlying principles are less important than the resulting achievement. Breaking the world into "atomistic, flexible" parts that can be reordered leads to rapid innovation. This efficiency is utterly intertwined with pragmatism. Pragmatic modularity created the assembly line and makes management possible (Hall and Lindholm 1999, 85–86). Linguist Jackendoff argues that modularity is fundamental to the cognitive organization of thought, organizing perception, emotion, and intersubjective communication (1996, 71–76).

The fundamental logics of biomedicine and alternative medicine are radically different. Evidence-based biomedicine is a stochastic science, based on statistical probabilities derived from clinical trials. Information is compiled on diseases, etiologies, interventions, and the collective characteristics of a population. Only the variables under consideration, such as a measurable change in symptom following a pharmaceutical intervention, are relevant. The totality of circumstances in a particular person's life is not under consideration. The basic assumption is that experimental treatment variables can be disaggregated from the whole person, manipulated, and measured to yield new knowledge about particular therapies that can then be applied to any member of the appropriate population to achieve the same result. In a larger sense, biomedicine has been increasingly statistical since the mid-eighteen hundreds. Health was *normalized*—that is, made progressively more statistical and defined as the *measurable* absence of disease (Warner 1997, 94). Physicians turned away from viewing health as a natural, almost metaphysical state. Numbers became the basis for decision-making, interpretation, and communication. The use of statistics becomes the appropriate mechanism for making prognoses, which are, after all, derived from the measurements of clinical trials (Kaufman 2005, 47). Statisticians count the number of people with a particular disease who have a specific demographic profile. They also track the length of survival for patients with a specified intervention.

Holistic alternative healing practices are based on entirely different premises. In naturalistic medical systems, each person is a unique configuration of inherent constitutions, relationships, environments, and attitudes that look beyond the physically knowable world.[3] The efficacy of a therapy cannot be generalized to others in a statistical fashion. Only individual trial and error can demonstrate empirically whether a remedy will work. Instead of statistical inference, the only valid standard is whether or not the remedy works on that particular person. If it worked on a family member or friend, that constitutes evidence that a remedy or practice might be worth trying. Such "anecdotal" evidence is suggestive of efficacy, but only direct experimentation by the person will reveal whether that intervention will help that particular person in that specific environment (English-Lueck 1990, 74–75). The experiential side of health, the qualitative *sensation* of vitality and wellness, is the metric that matters. We see one measure of wellness repeatedly cited: *energy*. A person's feeling of energy and productive vitality translates directly into interpreting oneself as healthy.

The conflict between the quantitative and qualitative metrics of health can be seen in how menopause is constructed in each epistemology. Women aging into their fifties are experiencing the quandary of menopause management. Is it a hormonal deficiency disease where the reduction of estrogen and testosterone can be measured and "corrected" with appropriate medication (see McCrea 2003)? Or is it a natural condition to be felt, experienced, and managed by changes in diet, exercise, and herbal modulation? Debbie Carson, having already experienced the surgical removal of her ovary and uterus, experimented with herbal remedies but felt herself becoming less mentally acute. She comments, "My mind just disappeared!" She had her hormones tested and went on low-dose testosterone therapy, in addition to the herbal interventions she was already employing. Debbie used two different metrics that combined numerical data with experiential knowledge to reach a decision that worked for her. Each diagnostic logic and corresponding therapy constitutes a module. It was more important to Debbie that the treatments worked for her, in ways she could trust and understand, than that their medical rationales were fundamentally different.

Jean Sanders uses slightly different metrics to make her decision. In her early fifties her physician wanted her to take "estrogen. I was really reluctant; fearful about cancer. She gave me good reasons, that it would preserve mental ability and bones, and at this time, I was beginning to suffer hot flashes." Jean was warned that she would need to continue hormone replacement therapy or suffer bone loss. However, her **chiropractor** used muscle testing to monitor her hormones and told her that it was not estrogen she needed, but progesterone. Jean comments, "That made sense to me since [estrogen] is stored in body fat—of which I have no shortage!" The chiropractor recommended a cream that used "natural hormones" derived from wild yam, to be rubbed directly onto the breasts, abdomen, and thighs. It can be found in health food chain stores. After she attended a workshop at her worksite on menopause and discovered others using the cream, she was encouraged. She continued using the cream until she completed menopause. While attending to the chemical side of the experience, she also grappled with the emotional side. She had no intention of having more children, yet she experienced "a loss of fertility. I viewed it as a loss, the end of that stage of my life." She missed the rhythm of menstrual periods, saying, "I feel flat. You get used to the sun going up and down, and the loss of the cycle is initially difficult to get used to," but she ultimately harmonized with her new life stage. Her view of it as natural, in line with her spiritual and political values, allowed her to use a metric other than laboratory tests to measure hormonal deficiency.

Measured and Experienced, Rival Metrics

Navigating the quantitative and qualitative metrics that connect different health frameworks is a necessary skill in deep medical diversity. Even though the epistemological underpinnings of naturalistic medicine and biomedicine are radically different, they merge in everyday use. Debbie Carson's experience is increasingly like that of patients in contemporary China, where the choice of traditional Chinese medicine, *zhongyi*, or Western biomedicine, *xiyi*, is available to many urban dwellers. People choose medical options based on the "recognized features of the different systems in relation to their specific illnesses or illness episodes, knowledge, previous experiences, and other practical concerns, such as cost or convenience" (Zhang 2007, 17). In China, for example, *zhongyi* and *xiyi* evolved along separate lines. *Zhongyi* is seen as a humanistic tradition that does not uncouple people from the natural world the way analytical scientific medicine does. Nonetheless, considerable effort has been put into scientizing *zhon-gyi* (see ibid., 28). Using the language of clinical tests and numeric metrics lends modernist cultural authority to traditional practices. Similarly, some American acupuncturists cite a measurable endorphin release in defense of their method for pain management. Nearly every naturalistic diet, ranging from vegetarianism to raw foods, mentions measurable weight loss as a benefit in addition to the restoration of vitality.

The practice of ChiRunning illustrates the complementary use of this dual metric system. ChiRunning, along with **ChiWalking**, is the invention of Danny and Katherine Dreyer. Looking for a way to reduce injury, they applied the principles of *taiji* to the practice of running. Citing Stephen Covey, author of the *Seven Habits of Highly Effective People*, they developed principles "that will help you to run, and train, in a more effortless and efficient way" (Dreyer and Dreyer 2004, 29). They apply the subtle bodily disciplines of *taiji* to the act of running: by focusing the mind, sensing the body, being aware of breath, relaxing and strengthening parts of the body. The body is held in alignment, head tall, knees soft. ChiRunners are taught to "zip their jeans"—that is, tightening the lower abdominal muscles, the *tandian*, to shift the impact of running from the delicate knees to the strong abdominal core. Running happens naturally as the person tilts forward and catches the body in erect posture; the legs are not pumped in front of the torso. The ChiRunner's arms are not rigid, swinging like pistons. Instead the arms are "soft," and swing gently behind the body. The lower back is kept flexible, but the core is stable, directing all motion forward, and minimizing unnecessary side-to-side motion. Running on a treadmill, or while plugged into an Apple iPod, is discouraged; distractions take the runner's awareness away from natural *qi*. The runner should enhance *qi* energy by concentrating inward on breath and outward observing nature; sufficient rest and healthful food also restore *qi*. Bay Area ChiRunning trainers are sensitive to the needs of older clients who want to run but are timid about injuring their wearable parts. Protecting knees, backs, and hips is of paramount concern. Yet ChiRunning is also supported by quantitative metrics that validate and support it. Biomechanical efficiency is enhanced by counting. ChiRunning is best done to a metronome, carefully set to eighty-five to ninety beats per minute (ibid., 82–83).

During the ChiRunning training, I took my own full-figured, fifty-four-year-old body around the parking lot of a sporting goods store, along with the rest of the class. In response to a question about weight-loss, Cliff, our trainer, explains that ChiRunning is too efficient to be used as a weight management system; it doesn't burn enough calories. Instead, persons needing to lose weight need to rethink their relationship with food. After saying this, he fixed me with a penetrating look—or so I felt at the time. Do I use food as a source of *qi,* a connection to nature, or as an addictive source of emotional comfort? As the group runs, Cliff corrects our postures, gives quantitative hints—for example, to concentrate on each component for one full minute before moving awareness to another component. Cliff explains that some of his trainees need the science and math to motivate them to practice, while other clients quickly become aware of the flow of energy and the lack of pain. Cliff reiterates that children "naturally" run this way. It is not until coaches and parents emphasize winning and speed that they push themselves into injury. Throughout the training, Cliff moves back and forth between drawing on quantitative metrics of bioefficiency to ways of discerning "nature" and the subjective metaphysics of *qi.*

Pamela Ibarra and Joan Linden, Watching Their Numbers

Nowhere is the dance of quantitative and qualitative explanations more evident than in the discourses about eating. Decades ago, anthropologists de la Rocha and Lave investigated the **ethnomathematics** of food consumption. Food can be translated into measurable calories, grams of fiber, sodium, carbohydrates, and nutrients, and thus viewed as overwhelmingly quantitative. Systems of weight management, such as **Weight Watchers**, simplify the calculation of nutritional value by providing an alternative system of points—using a formula that converts the number of calories, and the amounts of fat and fiber to a single number. Watching people using this system, de la Rocha discovered that people found ways to convert the constant need to measure the food to direct experience. Instead of measuring the food into one graduated cup, these women fill the container to the level of a particular design in the bowl itself and create a new set of intuitive visual cues (de la Rocha 1986, 139; de la Rocha 1985, 194; Lave 1996, 92). People learn to convert numbers into feelings of satisfaction and fullness, and that helps them internalize the meaning of the measurements.

Pamela Ibarra converts the "legal" foods allowable in the Weight Watchers program into practices she can incorporate into her life. She cannot bear to throw food out, and eating half a banana seems wasteful to her, so she adjusts her diet using her Weight Watchers book of points as a guide. Pamela eats legal foods such as celery, carrots, and beets to achieve a feeling of satiety before she goes to a special event. She has learned to drink coffee to get energy and fullness, to take away that "wanting to eat right away" feeling. She has quantitative and qualitative goals. She wants to lose thirty more pounds, but she also wants to stave off diabetes and "just feel good." Although her fasting glucose is 89 (within normal range), Pamela has **neuropathy**—numbness in her toes—and a family history of diabetes. That combination has alarmed her physician, who has given her a **glucometer** and a prescription for Glucophage, a medication for diabetes.

Joan Linden would weep with joy to have Pamela's laboratory test numbers. Younger than Pamela by a decade, Joan struggles with her diabetes. She loathes her glucometer, because it symbolizes her struggle to get her blood glucose under control. She exercises devoutly, eats a lacto-ovo vegetarian diet, which allows milk and egg products, and measures her blood glucose and takes insulin. Her numbers, however, remain high, and Joan laments, "I can have the perfect little breakfast and have taken a nice long walk and check it and it's like, 'Oh, fuck, it's 273,' you know." She is frustrated that this number dominates her interactions with the medical system. Joan admires her endocrinologist but jokingly relates, "You know, my doctor—God bless her," when she sees her, "It's not like, 'How are you?' It's like, 'Did you bring your meter in? What's your [number]'? I could send my meter and not send myself in sometimes, you know, that's how it feels. . . . I couldn't come today, but my meter could come!" Medical efficiency demands that numbers be the language of patient-therapist communication, but Joan wants to express herself as something more.

Joan's frustration is in part because she herself is deeply immersed in another way of looking at the world. Her house is a blend of Catholic and

Tibetan Buddhist imagery. Her husband teaches Buddhism and she is a hospice counselor. Spirit and feeling are not distant abstractions, but part of her everyday world. In contrast to the numbers, she says, "I think my energy level is another metric. . . . 'I don't have energy for this' or 'Oh, I'm really tired.'" Another "metric" for her, although she has a hard time putting it into words, is her "grief with it," her frustrations at the mismatch between her own approach and that of biomedicine. "I think there's another part of me. . . . I feel so pissed off." The American Diabetes Association diet definitely does not have her in mind. She is not interested in meat or fancy desserts. She is angry at her meter, upset with the "manipulation" of companies who provide glucometers for free but charge a fortune for the test strips. She does not feel "well supported by her insurance" and feels the pinch of every purchase. However, she has a "pre-existing condition," which limits her coverage and choices.

So she experiments with alternatives. She tried a concoction of juiced vegetables from local Asian markets and pig's pancreas, and it helped for a few months. She takes alpha-lipoic acid and uses Rick Mendosa's local website—he has since moved to Colorado—to vet a number of alternative and biomedical practices related to diabetes. She is determined to understand the role of cortisol, a hormone that signals the liver to release more glucose. Cortisol is related to stress and is an emotive metric she *can* understand. Stress is a commonly understood etiology for ordinary people with the disease (Schoenberg et al. 2005).

Accommodating the two systems of knowing is one of the greatest challenges facing this aging cohort. In studying a group of men in a Veterans Hospital, ranging in age from their fifties to their eighties, medical anthropologist Ferzacca heard a common refrain: "By me, it's going okay. By the records, it's not so good" (Ferzacca 2000, 33). Making sense of the competing metrics is vital to the project of managing self and aging well.

Jean Sanders, Restaging Middle Age, Aging Well

This concept, "aging well," is part of a larger narrative that questions the cultural assumptions of life staging. The popular construct reflects a new biomedical vision of "**health span**" as opposed to mere "lifespan," in which "the onset of age-related diseases" can be held at bay (Rattan and Clark 2005, 297). Health span, as a term, is rooted in gerontological discourse aimed at reducing the progressive accumulating of molecular damage experienced as aging. However, the term also embraces the psychosocial, referring to extending the period of productivity rooted in cognitive abilities and social functioning (Miriam Lueck, Institute for the Future, personal communication, July 3, 2008). While the physical consequences of aging cannot be denied, even by the most fit and augmented of this age cohort, the notion that age needs to be disabling is being questioned. The most wealthy and educated of this cohort assert the probability of longevity, while denying the inevitability of decrepitude and nonproductivity. Instead, using the tools of self-invention, they prepare for a different experience of aging than that undergone by their parents.

Jean Sanders, who is nearly the same age as Enduring Pine's Sofia, articulately expresses the philosophy of aging well and converts words to practices. She thinks of health as vigor, energy, and the "power to do what I want to do!" After marrying, divorcing, and raising her now-adult sons, she is retiring from her admin job to pursue a doctorate. For her entire adult life she has had skin problems, autoimmune conditions such as eczema and **psoriasis**, osteoporosis, and arthritis. The psoriasis is particularly painful in her feet. Over the last five years the problems have become more acute, and she has had to rethink her future. Jean reflects, "Studies show that it's likely that I'm going to live into my nineties. I don't have enough income to really survive those long numbers of years without a good career with good income. Working is probably not only something I want to do—because I have a lot of energy for it—but it's also going to be necessary. So there's kind of a dual motivation there for me to look for another career."

While she had a stable job before retirement, with good benefits, it was not lucrative. That worries her. As she drives through Palo Alto she notes, "It's easy to identify—when you look at older people—who has money and who doesn't have money. You can tell by the way they walk how much pain they are in." She reflects, "When you have the financial resources to age well . . . it's easier to age well. It's tragic that that should make such a difference, that people don't receive the health care that they need as they age. It looks terribly distressful." The fear such observations generate helped Jean to "shape my own decisions that I was making in my midlife, to begin to take some steps to start really taking care of myself and health." She knows it is possible because "I've had some wonderful role models, people in their eighties who are so alive and exciting. They are still contributing, and they are still sharing what they've learned. They're still working and active."

The narrative of healthy aging implies an alternative embodiment of life staging. Instead of viewing the aging process as the inevitable breakdown of the machine, the quality of aging is viewed as a personal choice. How one's body ages is the end product of specific decisions. Notice that the cultural narrative of the oldest age cohort is a curious mixture of metaphors of nature and manufacture. The body is simultaneously "naturally" decaying, while at the same time the machine metaphor invokes another sort of breakdown, one that is mechanical. A third, more subtle metaphor involved in the narrative of aging is "cradle to grave." This metaphor suggests that the person is like a consumer product chain, proceeding from conception to inevitable planned obsolescence.

In the revised conception of aging well, different components of body, behavior, and cognition can be sustained, replaced, or recycled, just as the design metaphor of "cradle to cradle" implies that the lives of products can be rethought, extended, and eventually recycled (McDonough and Braungart 2002). For example, a book created in the "cradle-to-grave" philosophy would make tree-derived paper; make the paper briefly into a book, and then leave the aging paper to decay. A cradle-to-cradle book could be made from synthetic materials—plastic resins and inorganic fibers. After its incarnation as a book the mock paper could be broken down into its component materials. Those materials can be remade into other products repeatedly. The "book" is designed from the onset to be sustainably reborn. Similarly, the metaphor of **sustainability** is being applied to the bodies of those who would age well.

This open-ended redesign metaphor is not limited to the physical body. Silicon Valley people repeatedly use aspects of neurolinguistic programming to reframe the language by which one thinks about oneself, enhancing the ability to reshape thought as well as action. Healthy aging is itself a mantra that recasts the conception of the experience. In the healthy aging framework, the person—body and mind—is assumed to be more sustainable with proper care. That care is partly biomedical—a life augmented with knee prosthetics, biological cancer therapies derived from genetically modified monoclonal antibodies, pacemakers, and insulin pumps—and yet deeply rooted in valuing the natural. Cleansing the environment and body of toxins, embracing physical movement, spiritual growth, and "real food" that has not been processed is also seen as innate to the stewardship of the self. The tools of productivity—management and goal-direction—are harnessed to facilitate this healthy aging.

Jean's nearly crippling psoriasis in her feet threatened to disrupt her life because she "couldn't walk very easily . . . knowing that walking is a really important part of maintaining the rest of my body." She consults podiatrists, dermatologists, Ayurvedic practitioners, acupuncturists, and herbalists. Jean develops "a very complex [system] of using the various things" she had been told to do by different practitioners. "Through a process of trial and error" she balances her various modular practices so that her chronic conditions will not go "out of control." If she doesn't "adhere to the program . . . the pain returns" and she needs to get "back on track." Each morning Jean moves through what she calls her "practice." She performs a set of exercises designed to limber her body, many gleaned from twenty years of yoga. She lifts weights, she prays, and does *zazen* Buddhist meditations. She elevates her feet for ten to twenty minutes out of every hour. She takes vitamins. It is more difficult to remember her Fosamax, since that osteoporosis medication is taken only once a week. She sets up a reminder on her computer the night before and sets the bottle next to her coffee pot for Sunday morning. These daily practices form the foundation of her health management regime and jump-start her day. Jean observes, "I love waking up feeling good, and I'm excited about life."

She compares this experience of experimentation to the excitement of raising her sons: "It's that transforming." Daily practices are embedded in longer, more daring experiments. Jean has created cohesive modules, six-month forays into particular alternative therapies to help her manage her chronic ills. For example, Jean "found a medical doctor that had studied Ayurvedic medicine, the traditional medical system of India, and he prescribed a particular diet. I adhered to it precisely. It was the best adherence that I've ever accomplished in my life. It was such a big change for me. I was in so much pain and so desperate, and I thought that maybe this could work." She used herbs and ointments directly on her feet, and altered her diet to include rabbits, catfish, and other Ayurvedic "cooling foods." With the help of her partner she scoured the region looking for ingredients, because the Ayurvedic diet didn't "fit with anything in this country." However, together they found just the right kind of South Asian butcher shop—one advantage of living amid deep medical diversity—and she stuck to it long enough to assess that it was only partially successful for her. In the end, Jean reflects, "I could never tell whether it was helping or not." Acupuncture was more successful for her, and so it had a longer period of experimentation. Jean wove together short daily efforts with sustained multicultural trials into a hybrid and customized set of practices. As Ron Little suggested, practices have to be practical to be sustainable, but living in deeply diverse Silicon Valley expands the definition of what is realistic experimentation.

Jean's practices also included significant cognitive effort. A decade earlier, her son, Dennis, had been involved in a serious Jet Ski accident in which he was run over by a boat and nearly died. His response to that accident "really shaped my view of the health world." It was three weeks before she could bring Dennis to California on an airplane, and he spent months more in a bed in the kitchen. Jean remembers, "What I learned from Dennis, and why I think he was so successful in his healing, is that he took charge of it. . . . When the physical therapists came and worked with him, and they told him what to do, he did all of those things." Every day there was visible progress. "I could just see the healing happening before my eyes, and I think he could see it too. . . . We really focused on the healing, not on how bad it really was at that point. We would find something that he was healing, and we worked with our language . . . not calling it the 'bad leg.' It wasn't bad or good. We talked about the 'hurt leg.'" Dennis's attitude is another example of neuro-linguistic programming. "Somebody introduced us to a book . . . of visualizing himself healthy. He actively imagined himself getting well and getting better. I think that really positive attitude really contributed to his healing, and it also really contributed to his motivation to be compliant and adhere to what the doctors and therapists were telling him to do." Watching Dennis create his practices for healing inspired Jean in her healthy aging strategy: "That was instructive for me, too. I'm sure I'm applying some of that now."

Jean uses a number of **affirmations** to reprogram her thinking, such as: " 'My muscles are strong and supple.' 'I feed myself appropriately and make good decisions for myself.' 'My mind is focused and conscious.' 'My immune system is strong and powerful. It protects my healthy cells and doesn't mistakenly attack them.' 'My skin and bones and toes are normal and healthy.' I just keep those thoughts going through my head while I'm doing this whole practice." Jean is not alone in her self-reformation; her family was part of her ecology of beliefs and practices. Her openness to particular philosophies influences her sons, and they, in turn, inspire her. Jean illustrates a number of lessons about the first wave. She is experimental, borrowing and testing practices from her deeply medically diverse region. These practices come in thought and action modules that can be mixed, adapted, and customized to her needs. She stays focused on managing her emerging chronic illnesses, but with the positive goal of aging well. Jean Sanders uses her intelligence and resources to accomplish that objective. Even though Jean is the agent of those changes, she does not establish the goals or accomplish them alone. She works within a web of kin and fictive kin that help her.

Debbie Carson, Families Feeling Capitalism

Families, not just individuals, adopt and enact particular strategies for self-care and health management. People in the first wave are famously sandwiched between competing familial obligations, managing care for three generations—for their parents, their children, and themselves as they age. As health care becomes increasingly fragmented, American families, especially the caretaker mothers, are "empowered" to make more decisions on their own. The marketplace for defining health—biomedical, diverse, and alternative—is difficult to manage, and families must develop strategies to navigate it. Debbie Carson—married to Martin Kline, the mother of Ethan and Derek Rogers—has learned to apply her expertise as a former high-technology purchaser to the task. She manages Ethan's **ADHD**—attention deficit hyperactivity disorder—and other ailments, using a combination of biomedical and naturopathic practices. She has also inadvertently taught her sons a health management strategy that mirrors her own.

According to Debbie, Ethan was an endlessly restless child, always flitting from thing to thing. Debbie suspected ADHD, but Jason Rogers, her first husband and Ethan's and Derek's father, disagreed. That was one of the issues of contention when they divorced. Debbie took Ethan to child psychiatrists at the HMO, and he was placed on the first of a series of medications that would continue through his adolescence into college. But he was never on Ritalin, the most popular medication for boys with his diagnosis. Debbie distrusted the information coming from Ciba-Geigy, the pharmaceutical company that made the drug, and as the support groups and medical practitioners were given the same information, they too became suspect. Fine-tuning his medication was a constant challenge. At one point he was on Prozac and sleeping twenty-three hours a day; he was unable to function. He missed six weeks of school and a European vacation with his grandparents. The HMO lost his test results, and Debbie's patience dwindled. Finally Debbie took him to her naturopathic practitioners, and they told her to drop his medication: "Now!" She responded, "But I can't. You know the doctors." They disagreed, telling her, "Take him off! Take him off!" She did. After Ethan's dramatic improvement Debbie reflected, "Once again, it was a huge instance where Western medication totally fried us—and Eastern medication didn't." By mixing her epistemological modules, she crafted a therapeutic path for Ethan.

Debbie's strategies for caring for Ethan are illustrated by another incident. He had mononucleosis, and, faced with a teen "falling apart," Debbie had to discern the cause of her son's exhaustion. The physician at the HMO initially denied it was mono, but her naturopath, Kari, disagreed and insisted that he should be tested. Her trust in Kari far exceeds her trust in biomedicine. Debbie comments, "As the years have gone on, I've gotten to the point that I trust her far more than I trust doctors, because she will sit and talk to me for two hours, if that's what it takes." Since the HMO had entrusted her with a lab slip, Debbie filled it out to test for Epstein-Barr specific antibodies, and it was positive. Armed with this diagnosis, she returned to the HMO for his treatment. Each phase of the medical encounter—suspecting an illness, testing, diagnosis, and treatment—was drawn from multiple medical paradigms, minute medical modules open to negotiation and reshuffling. Debbie Carson, on behalf of her youngest son, has become a master navigator of medical institutions.

Debbie also manages her parents' health care. They live in another state, and Debbie does all the health care work that involves research or purchasing online, because her mother "is afraid that the gray box is going to eat her. I mean, she gets her email and that's about it—that's all she'll do with it." Debbie looks up information on particular diagnoses or pharmaceuticals, prints it out, and then faxes the pages to her mother. Her technological savvy became critical when her parents' health care insurance coverage changed. Debbie relates, "They had what they thought was a really good health plan, and in January [the providers] dropped all prescription coverage . . . just left all of these seniors out high and dry. . . . They were faced with a $450 bill [for prescription drugs]." Debbie explains, "They've done a lot of make-shift things." They have been stockpiling samples, "because they knew that this was coming. They found out in September that they were going to be dropped [from coverage] in January, so they started to move their prescriptions up by a week or two, to start stockpiling things." Debbie then came to the rescue, investigating the mechanism by which she could get drugs from Canada, getting all the documentation, faxing it to the right people, and ordering online for her parents.

Debbie's health history is complex. Many of these diagnoses come from her encounters with biomedicine. She had an ovarian cyst removed, but that complicated her experience with menopause. When her husband, Martin, was working in Europe, she visited him and picked up a persistent foot fungus. She too has been diagnosed with ADHD, is clinically depressed, and struggles with her weight. She has been diagnosed with two syndromes that are poorly received within biomedicine—chronic fatigue and multiple chemical sensitivities. Years of pain led to chemical dependency on prescription pain medications, although she is proud to state that she has been "clean and sober for eight years." Now her primary provider of care is a naturopath who is learning traditional Chinese medicine and has earned her trust. So Debbie copes with an alternative "diagnosis," low kidney fire, a deficiency of the **kidney meridian**, a channel for *qi*. Her daily medical regime can include up to a hundred pills a day, including homeopathic remedies, vitamins, Chinese herbs, and biomedical pharmaceuticals. Each therapy is researched, documented, and its effect recorded by Debbie. Her computer and photocopier are seldom idle.

Medical anthropologists have noted that multiple chemical sensitivity is a socially problematic category. In California, 6.3 percent report a diagnosis of environmental illness, and 15.9 percent report being "allergic or highly sensitive to everyday chemicals." Moreover, there is no clear test for people with MCS; blood counts, urinalysis, EKGs, and so forth are usually normal. Pharmaceuticals can make symptoms worse, rather than better (Lipson 2004, 202–8). The mechanism for the disease's etiology and manifestation is unclear. Rather than clearly responding to measurable chemical amounts—the levels of chemical contamination to which people react are often below that now considered the safe-unsafe threshold—people sort themselves into categories of nonsensitive, sensitive, and "hypersensitive" bodies. This is an approach that doesn't work well for biomedicine (Kroll-Smith and Floyd 1997, 20). The illness produces invisible disabilities, which are often relegated by biomedical practitioners to "the mind," and therefore the malady becomes the exclusive burden of the individual to manage. Most baffling to physicians is the "body's increasing intolerance to ordinary, putatively benign places and mundane consumer products" (ibid., 19). People with MCS are likely to create a regimen in which they avoid triggers, rather than seek drugs or other invasive medical therapies (ibid., 21). Outwardly healthy people cannot go to a mall where people will be wearing fragrances and where the residue of cleaning chemicals is all around. Debbie can stay only in a hotel that has guaranteed nonsmoking rooms—which excludes much of the world—and by bringing in her own cleaning supplies. Martin, her husband, will come in first, clean the room, and air it out. Then, perhaps, she can enter it without having blinding migraines and bodily pain. Workplaces can be similarly problematic.

Debbie left her lucrative job in high-tech purchasing for a semiconductor firm when it became clear that should chemicals leak from the clean room she would feel it within minutes. Like other people with multiple chemical sensitivities, she calls herself the "canary in the coal mine," linking her microcosmic self to macrocosmic environmental degradation. Passionately, Debbie asserts, "We're poisoning our systems, we're poisoning our bodies—we're poisoning our air and our water, and I'm one of those people who react to it first. Lucky me." She changed her career and became a historical interpreter; she feels safe in older, preindustrial buildings. She had to quit one job, however, when the museum in which she worked was remodeled. Such incidents are common to people with MCS (Lipson 2004, 206). Debbie found the paint and glue fumes unbearable. She monitors her environment closely and uses specialized soaps and paints. She educates her family and friends to avoid scented cosmetics and arms herself with an array of nonscented products—low-toxicity new materials that do not off-gas. Air-filters and masks, bought from Lab Safety and Supply, limit her inhalation of organic vapors. There is little or no institutional support for her disability, but she puts together a collage of practices that mitigates her distrust of biomedicine's motives and enhances her access to alterative resources. Debbie consciously tracks her many medical modules and comfortably employs any combination that will work for her. She is an "empowered" health consumer.

Debbie Carson builds her own customized assemblage of health information modules. She uses the "objective knowledge" provided by biomedical laboratory diagnoses and the statistically informed clinical trials that validate her medications. She pushes the system to give her medications outside of the standard **formulary** of her provider, the list of drugs the organization may prescribe without additional justification. Her use of a spare laboratory test form, which she used for her son Ethan, is another example of asserting agency to navigate the bureaucracy of the provider.

Debbie understands the different logics of the several medical systems she uses as modules in her larger health care ecosystem. She uses alternative diagnostic procedures, such as muscle testing, as well as biomedical ones. Muscle testing is a naturopathic method of determining whether a particular substance is good for that unique individual. The substance in question is held on the body while arms or legs are held out. In order to "test" the muscle, the therapist will bear down and measure the strength of resistance. The greater the client's strength, the more benign is the substance. Other forms of alternative diagnosis can also be used: examining the tongue, the eyes, and the general shape of the body. The practitioner watches how the person moves, listens for her emotional expression, and tracks her behavior patterns. The naturopath then infers underlying energy and emotional patterns. This discovery is followed by the appropriate intervention—such as an herbal concoction or pill, a homeopathic remedy, a change in diet, or new behavioral practice.

Debbie does not limit her therapeutic process to one medical epistemology. There is no simple sequence, such as that suggested decades ago by sociologist Talcott Parsons, in which the "patient" experiences symptoms, decides she is ill, goes to a doctor, accepts the diagnosis and follows the recommended treatment, tracks symptoms, and adheres to all of the required bureaucratic procedures (Falcon and Spalding 2004, 15; Gabe, Bury, and Elston 2004, 91–96; James and Hockey 2007, 29). Rather, each step of this process is weighed using different criteria of risk, informed by trust, experience, and political philosophy. There are many modular market alternatives for diagnosis, treatment, measurement, tracking, and provisioning. Imagine that instead of one linear process, there are many modules, each drawing on different medical epistemologies from which a person may choose at any stage of the process. The deep medical diversity of the San Francisco Bay Area makes the complexity and potential conflicts of the modules only more evident. The final outcome—health and well-being—is more important than maintaining one consistent underlying philosophy.

The fact that Martin, Debbie's husband, has good work-based insurance facilitates Debbie's access to pharmaceuticals. Her OB-GYN at the HMO works with Kari, the naturopath, to explore combinations of herbal concoctions and hormonal therapies. Martin can get a more concentrated version of Debbie's Chinese medications when he is in The Netherlands, which adds to her locally purchased supply of herbal pills. Eco-friendly, low-toxicity products are easily available for her, since the San Francisco region is a center for green health. While Debbie's decisions are shaped by her visceral distrust of biomedicine and her strong physical reaction against eco-hostile materials, she experiments with options regularly with *materia medica* drawn from different philosophies. Debbie is a competent master of modularity. The intimacy of alternative practice draws Debbie. At other times, the efficiency of biomedicine is useful. She uses the former to act as a check on the latter, using herbal remedies to regulate the impact of pharmaceuticals on her particular body.

Ethan and Derek Rogers, Learning at Their Mother's Knee

Ethan Rogers, Debbie's youngest son, plans to be an electrical engineer like his father, and eventually, he will fulfill this dream. Ethan knows that if he only studies math and science he'll become just another techno-geek, and he won't make the kind of impact he wants to make. To make a difference he must be a manager and begin to build a life of civic engagement. Through watching the actions of his parents' generation he knows such a path requires careful crafting. So he consciously and deliberately works on himself.

Tall, slender, with blond boyish charm, Ethan is a bit shy. He counteracts this "flaw" by performing in school plays, singing in the choir, and seeking opportunities to voice his opinion in his classes. He volunteers in the community, either through the school or to support his mother's efforts. When he goes off to college he plans to live with business majors, and not engineers, since they are more "outgoing and well rounded." Dale Carnegie's 1937 self-help classic, *How to Win Friends and Influence People* and Stephen Covey's 1989 *Seven Habits of Highly Effective People* are on his reading list.

In spite of his optimism and self-cultivation, Ethan has serious concerns about the way people's work seems to affect their lives. When Ethan reflects on the high levels of depression around him, he suggests that it is because of "the lack of social skills. . . . People sleep less in this area and people are less social because one of the things that comes with social skills . . . is the realization that working more than fifty hours a week is unhealthy—though physically possible, mentally and socially, you know, it's unhealthy. . . . I think sooner or later there will be a backlash against that." Nonetheless, Ethan believes the situation will improve, not by resisting work itself but through the efficiencies of "the technology that evolves during our generation," which will lead to "spectacular changes."

During summer break he plans to work at Fry's Electronics, the iconic gadget superstore in the Silicon Valley, where he has shopped with his Dad since childhood. Ethan is wistful about his childhood. He has no recollection of his father saying, "I am a father," but only, "I am an engineer." Ethan reflects on his own future as a father—he once told his mother not to worry that he "will breed." He has laid out a parenting plan of his own. He hopes he will remember the finer points when he actually enacts his plan.

Derek Rogers, Ethan's elder brother, has chosen a deeply embodied profession, in spite of his strong family connection to information technology. Derek, a university student, is an actor in training, who must be intimately conscious of his own bodily movements, expressions, and voice qualities to perform on the stage. He is also the son of an engineer, stepson of an MIS (management and information services) accountant, and brother to an aspiring engineer. Even though he is an artist, he takes the Physics for Engineers course at the university rather than the lighter version offered to humanities students. His time spent in online chats is as much a part of his social life as the time in the green room before and after performances talking with the other actors. It is in this hybrid technological and humanistic context that Derek undertakes to manage his body. Actors routinely stretch, exercise, and do "integrated breaths." They box, breathe, and chant an e.e. cumming's poem, furiously scribbled by the watching anthropologist:

> my father moved through dooms of love
> through sames of am through haves of give,
> singing each morning out of each night
> my father moved through depths of height.

Derek is wiry, tall, and graceful but not "buff." His theatrical coach, a powerful African-American actor and director, undertakes special sessions in the gyms for the "skinny white boys" to give them muscular definition. He is exhausted, having slept only two hours the night before, working on his monologue and his almost-due ten-page paper. His housemates, almost all theater students, did not sleep at all. When they reach the gym, the three young men bench press fifty, ninety, and finally a hundred pounds. They move to weight machines designed to sculpt upper back, chest, and shoulders. His legs have already been injured from his dance class, in preparation for an upcoming musical, and he dare not risk injuring them further by joining his classmates in leg work.

Twice a week Derek goes to his mother's naturopath to work on the pain in his knees and hips. Derek moves effortlessly between biomedicine, which, like his mother, he does not entirely trust, and alternative healing. He suffers nosebleeds and attributes them to taking Retin-A during his freshman year for acne, which "wrecked my body." He pours soy milk on his breakfast cereal. Derek is conscious of the power of emotions, and he works with the naturopath to strengthen his mind-body connection. Managing his sexuality is also part of the larger agenda of bodily experimentation, fitness, and control. He explores several relationships simultaneously, each one characterized by varying levels of seriousness, emotional risk, and different levels of sexual engagement.

Some families build consensus about the directions and limits of experimentation. Debbie Carson and her sons, Ethan and Derek, all enact a common frame of reference mediated by Kari, Debbie's naturopath. Even the Carson cat, Tristan, is treated with alternative veterinary medicine. Other families may be more internally diverse: vegetarians sharing Thanksgiving meals with turkey-eating carnivores; a Chinese wife who mystifies her Irish husband by excluding certain foods from her diet because they are forbidden to postpartum women. Families are already experimenting with deep medical diversity. As members of families and social networks engage in new practices, they become conduits of knowledge to others. Their experiences, whether constructive or disastrous, will shape further experimentation in the family.

The cohort born after World War II changed the way health was sought, aging was conceptualized, and work was done. Margaret Ginsberg illustrates many features of the Silicon Valley health culture that blended countercultural aspirations with technological optimism. Margaret, like Ron Little and Jean Sanders, experiments with language, the software of well-being, to consciously create an environment that supports wellness practices. Creeping into middle age, keeping healthy is an increasingly difficult proposition, as the wearable parts need care. The first wave experimenters employ distinctly alternative medical systems. Enduring Pine Healing Center provides a deeply diverse hybrid of classical Chinese medicine and countercultural experimentation to its clients, as does Kari, Debbie Carson's naturopath and Jean Sander's Ayurvedic practitioner. Alternative medical systems provide a language for qualitative assessments of health that complement, contextualize, and occasionally contend with quantitative biomedical understandings. Joan Linden would attest to the problematic dance of understanding her own chronic struggle with diabetes as both a set of biomedical metrics and a state of being. The cohort of the first wave were largely socialized into "traditional biomedicine" and came to complementary and alternative medicine as adults, and so create visibly hybrid practices that are then learned by younger generations. Debbie and Martin were raised with rather conventional notions about medicine, but Debbie's sons, Ethan and Derek, navigate multiple logics of heath seamlessly. Jean, Ron, and Margaret are determined to age well, to defy the assumptions about the life stage their parents embodied. To do so they have intertwined their health practices with work, the dominant force in their lives, which can alternatively support or subvert healthy living. The first wave cohort was instrumental in co-opting work places and fellow workers to support their health regimes. At the same time, employers have learned to maximize the efficiency of their high-value workers by keeping them healthy. The first wave cohort influenced the health and work culture that followed them, creating a second wave of change.

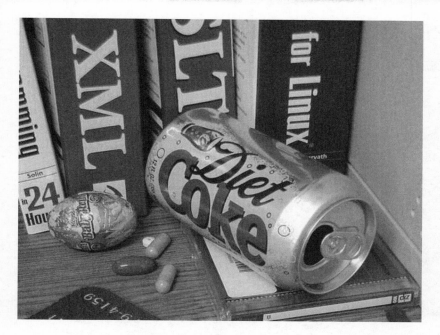

1. In Silicon Valley, caffeine, nutraceutical supplements, and sugar augment productivity. Photograph by J. A. English-Lueck.

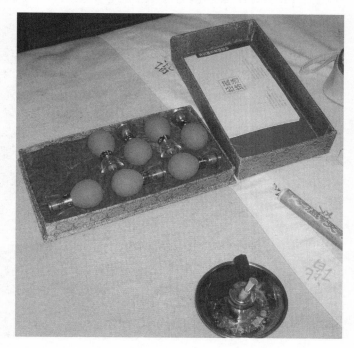

2. Celia, a practitioner of medical *qigong*, lays out the tools of her practice in her studio—including mugwort sticks for moxabustion and suction cups for cupping. Both techniques are used to effect change along the acupuncture meridians. Photograph by J. A. English-Lueck.

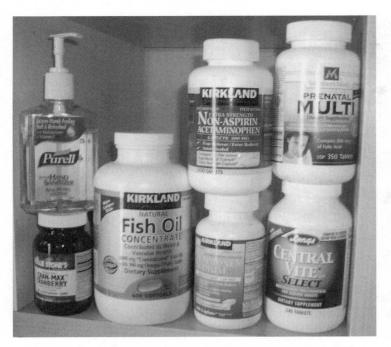

3. Like others in the second wave, Kristal and Jeremy use easily available supplements and functional foods to manage pain, hygiene, and preparation for eventual parenthood. Photograph by Richard Alvarado and Erin Dunham.

4. Kristal and Jeremy have consciously created an environment in their home to stay fit and healthy, especially now that they are both contingent workers. Jeremy tries to convince Kristal that DDR, Dance Dance Revolution, and the Wii are really fitness tools. Photograph by Richard Alvarado and Erin Dunham.

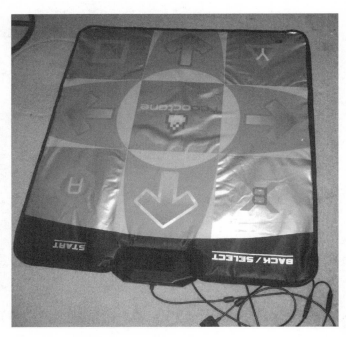

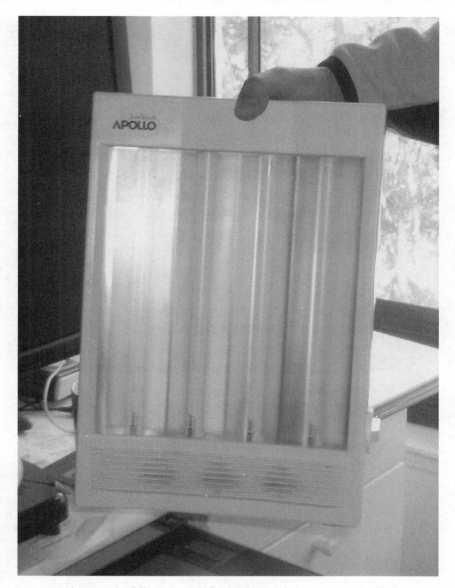

5. Jeremy shows us the full-spectrum light they keep to help manage Kristal's sleep problems and quest for energy. Her surgery for sleep apnea seems to be working, but nonetheless they maintain a strict separation between waking and sleeping. The lights reinforce daytime wakefulness, in contrast to the quiet isolated bedroom. Photograph by Richard Alvarado.

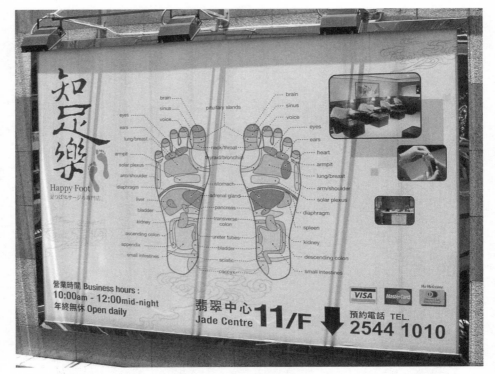

6. The intersection of traditional medicine and global holistic practices is not confined to Silicon Valley. In Hong Kong, foot reflexology is aimed at an international clientele. Photograph by J. A. English-Lueck.

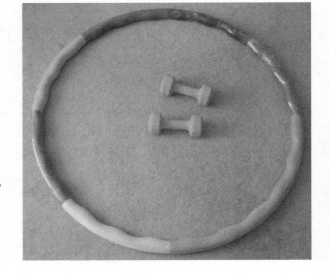

7. Addison has created an eco-system of exercise opportunities, at home and at work, to help her manage her weight. She will exercise up to five times a day. Photograph by Louise Ly.

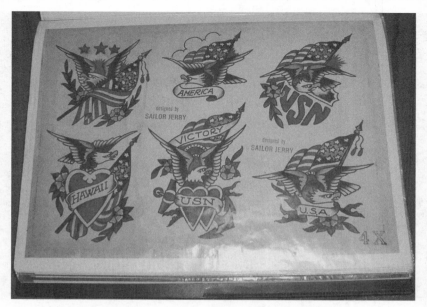

8. Flash, or standardized, tattoos are out of fashion, as they speak little about the "path" that person wants to inscribe upon his or her body. Photograph by J. A. English-Lueck.

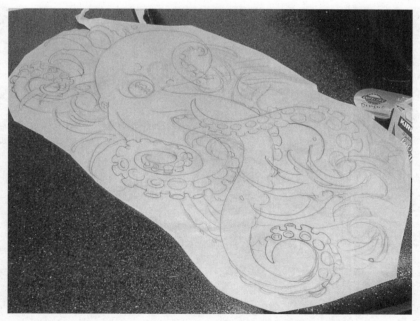

9. Working on identity can include body modification. Even that modification, however, is not necessarily permanent. Here Alan prepares a customized design that reworks a former design that no longer fits the client's self-image. Photograph by J. A. English-Lueck.

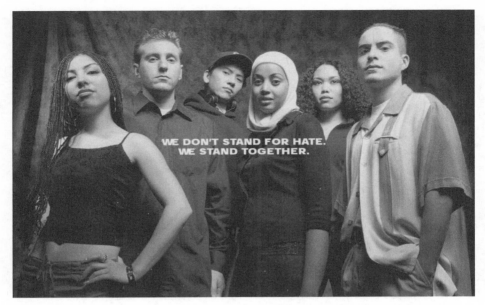

10. This poster, part of the Santa Clara County Network for a Hate-Free Community, creates an image of deep diversity and deep toleration. These values underpin the capacity to build deep medical diversity. Courtesy of Santa Clara County and Orloff/Williams.

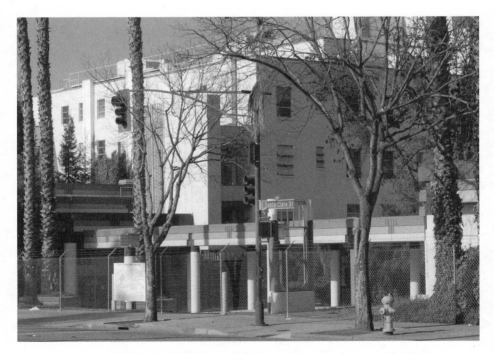

11. The San Jose Medical Center, which served the lower-income segments of the city center, closed in 2004. Photograph by Karl Lueck.

[handwritten notes, top of page:]

were dragging in full force for 2nd wave
→ neoliberalism – diminished benefits
health + retirement = innovation

- 'health as moral value' in the care
of others

3 In Produc...

definition

- new age beliefs reflect transcendentalism – environ...
as health +
- work as benefit to health ie resources +
community of support + draw on health   experimentation
- alternative medicine = crutch for capitalism?
- workplaces allies in wellness + family support? but why?

After planting, cutting, threshing, grinding the wheat and baking it into bread,
without the help of Pig, Cat and Rat, the little Red Hen asked,

"Who will eat the bread?" All the animals in the barnyard were watching
hungrily and smacking their lips in anticipation, and the Pig said, "I will," the
Cat said, "I will," the Rat said, "I will." But the Little Red Hen said, "No, you
won't. I will." And she did.

—Williams 2006, "The Little Red Hen," 24–25

- conferences of immigrants/
ethnic minorities looked into

Red hen on her side
flips dust under her wing
the free leg powerful
   levering leaves and dirt . . .

- field of parenthood + work
- turning to wellness programs = increase
efficiency + reduces health care
costs

May health, beauty,
Long life and wisdom
come to the barnyard fowl
   with humans to serve them:
World made for Red Hens.

—Snyder 1983, untitled poem, 53

recognizes impacts of work ethic on
capitalism

Kristal Jacobs and Jeremy Fitzgerald, Second Wave Workers

Second wave workers, such as Kristal Jacobs and Jeremy Fitzgerald, work
on their bodies to transform themselves into better workers, superior parents
and spouses, and, as they have come to define it, healthier people. Kristal and
Jeremy, both in their mid-thirties, occupy that liminal land of highly skilled,
self-employed **contractors**. Jeremy and Kristal are knowledge workers who
bring a specialized set of skills to workplaces. Jeremy has been a computer
programmer for five years, including a stint at a large CGI animation stu-

dio. Now he works independently and telecommutes from home. Kristal, his partner, also used to work with him in the East Bay. She is an ergonomics specialist who now contracts to various **web 2.0 companies** (organizations that specialize in hosted web services, social networking, wikis, blogs, and video sharing, such as eBay or Wikipedia). Their employers relate to them differently, with different obligations, as their status changes. A contract worker is not the same as an employee. Sometimes those distinctions can be happily navigated. Jeremy embraces the freedom his contract status gives him. Kristal is more hesitant; she no longer has access to the networks and resources she had as an employee. Jeremy and Kristal illustrate both the vulnerability that comes with contingent work and the experimental approach that second wave Silicon Valley workers so readily adopt.

For Jeremy, becoming a **contingent worker** turned his home into his workplace; the shift to telecommuting meant adopting a new set of disciplines. He no longer had the convenience of built in barriers between physically separate work and home spaces, and he needed to construct new ones. Jeremy notes, "You have to just create barriers for yourself. You have to say, 'Okay. I'm at home.' And even if you were really in the middle of something . . . at 7:00, 7:30, you're *done* with work. You need to eat, and then sort of wind down, and go to bed. You can't eat and then go back to work." The flip side of his new routine is even more challenging, "You have to get up in the morning, and sort of shower, put clothes on, shave, get in the right mindset. 'Okay. Now I'm doing work and not playing video games in the middle of the afternoon.'"

The new regime was also liberating. Work-home balance was a challenge at his last job. He reflects, "For a while, I was working sort of from the middle of the afternoon until four in the morning, trying to get this product finished. And it just wreaks havoc on your home life, your mental well-being. You just start to feel just not right. . . . I felt like I was sort of off-balance all the time." He found that it was hard to exercise, and yet "exercising is the only thing I found I could really do that at least helps somewhat."

In his newly redesigned routine, his life is increasingly local; Jeremy is "not really big on vacationing." He bikes, does a bit of rock climbing, and avidly plays soccer, although an old knee injury still causes him to favor one leg. Jeremy is conscious of growing older, but he has a plan. He designs a consistent routine, playing soccer regularly, and experimenting with running and other forms of activity "like . . . bicycling, lifting weights . . . various other cardio things. . . . I certainly need to have an exercise plan when I get older."

Jeremy knows that whatever he chooses, it must fit easily into the rest of his life, with as few obstacles as possible. In previous workplaces, there were onsite gyms and classes. Utilizing them only worked for him if their practices fit seamlessly into his life. He remembers, "I know that the first company I worked at had yoga classes, and so I went to the yoga classes. That's not something that I would necessarily do, but they had it there. . . . So I went. It was inexpensive, because the company was subsidizing it. I went, and it was good. . . . So when it was easy to do, I did it, and then, when it's not easy to do, I seem to not do it." Without the advantage of easy access, the effort taken to find special exercise sites is simply time spent away from home and work.

Jeremy and Kristal are conscious of the food they eat, the supplements they take, and the consequences of their consumption of liquid stimulants and relaxants. Jeremy cooks, institutes a daily practice of taking multivitamins, making sure that Kristal takes hers too (see Photograph 3). He will make a special effort to find good, fresh cuts of meat and brew good coffee. Stimulants hold a near-sacred place in the pantries of the second wave. Kristal comments, "We have every single coffee thing." They go out sometimes, and eat at the Indian and Chinese restaurants they favor, but they prefer one neighborhood sports bar just because it's fun. One of Jeremy's central tools for health is a nightly glass of wine at home. His father is a physician, and Jeremy draws on biomedical reasoning to explain his choices. He believes that red wine is good for older men, and yet he drinks it primarily for relaxation. Jeremy comments, "It sort of just relaxes you, and when you're relaxed, I think you feel better, and you're probably happy." Food and drink have functions, and those functions are consciously articulated as rationales for health practices.

Jeremy still uses his video games, but if he and Kristal play "Rayman Raving Rabbids" using the **Wii game console** three times a week they can actually move their bodies. In the game, they dash about holding their mobile nunchucks and drum for the dancing rabbits. Jeremy has been try-ing to win Kristal over to the world of gaming with Wii's "Dance Dance Revolution," claiming that it is really cardio exercise (see Photograph 4). Jeremy, more invested in the technological optimism and fascination that pervades Silicon Valley, tries to convert, or at least rationalize, his desire for digital gaming—a potentially deeply sedentary activity—with his need for exercise. Nintendo's Wii, a gaming system that requires some physical motion to play, helps him navigate this dilemma. Kristal wryly notes, "This is definitely a Silicon Valley solution for things."

Kristal is much more conscious of health than Jeremy, largely because she has struggled with a chronic condition much of her adult life. Kristal is thirty-four, a slightly overweight Eurasian woman who has hernias, sciatica, kidney stones, and ankle and knee injuries—four surgeries' worth. A car accident has left her in pain much of the time. Kristal has been tired since she was thirteen. This fatigue plagued her and mystified practitioners and only recently has been ameliorated. It was a constant struggle to get energy. Previous diagnoses led to medications that made her problems worse. She experiments with alternative products—"antioxidants, more cranberry, more pomegranate" to add energy. They drink Mango·Xan, a commercial energy tonic made from the Southeast Asian mangosteen fruit. Kristal's friend, Dee, whose husband is a chiropractor, is campaigning to wean her from over-the-counter anti-inflammatory medications.

Kristal has struggled with the amorphous and pervasive problem of fatigue, one that directly undermines her need for productivity. Weaving together diagnoses and practices from biomedicine and alternative medi-cine, she experiments on herself, much as Jean Sanders does with her pso-riasis. To boost their energy, Kristal and Jeremy use a sun lamp, "what they use in Sweden for people who are sunlight deprived to help get their bio-logical clock back. . . . But seriously, when we have trouble in winter time, we use this in the bedroom and turn it on in the morning to help us wake up." This appliance is one of the many devices the household members employ in their health ecosystem (see Photograph 5). Kristal reflects on her struggle with fatigue and comments, "I've lived with that all my life. So, we were just trying to get more energy in our days."

First diagnosed as depression and **narcolepsy**, her **sleep apnea** was finally pinpointed when she was thirty-two. Sleep apnea is a sleep disorder in which there are pauses in breathing during sleep. The consequences can be profound, ranging from irritability and memory loss to death. For a year and a half Kristal used a CPAP (continuous positive airway pressure) machine to blow air into her throat through a mask that was fitted over her nose. She sounded like Darth Vader and "looked like the thing that jumps out in Alien and grabs onto the guy's face." She slept as far from Jeremy as possible to keep from disturbing his sleep. Finally she had an operation to treat her obstructive sleep apnea—a maximal mandibular advancement surgically correcting the placement of her jaw. It was a difficult experience, and she gets support from her online sleepnet forum. Already Kristal can see the difference. She can get out of bed in the morning. Jeremy caught the flu and, for once, she did not get it! Her very emotions feel different to her—sharper. After a long series of medical and behavioral experiments, the results of the surgery appear promising to her.

With one problem resolved, Kristal tackles others. She knows she needs to change her overall "fat to lean muscle ratio." As a contractor, she does not have access to the gyms of her worksite. She will work on building muscle slowly and mindfully, approaching it as she does ergonomics; Kristal does not want just to solve the immediate physical problems, but to support her body for long-term change, including having children. Her goals are modest. Kristal says, "We don't need to be skin conscious, not be the people in the gym everyday. But be healthy, that means being outdoors, exercising, and eating well." Together, Jeremy and Kristal have experimented with a set of practices that are constantly being modified by trial and rejection, or trial and integration.

Second Wavers, Establishing Work and Family

People like Jeremy and Kristal, from their mid-twenties through their forties, are the cohorts that compose the primary workforce of Silicon Valley. These second wave workers are "in production." Employees and entrepreneurs juggle career, family, civic consciousness, and health. From their quarter-life crises to their midlife crises, they not only form the critical core of the productive workforce but also must imagine and build families, struggle with fading youth, and navigate the public and private bureaucracies that dominate American life. People in this age group must navigate the dual moral imperatives of keeping themselves and their families healthy and applying the work ethic to their careers.

Their immediate elders in the first wave defied conventional wisdom about the life staging of work. Americans imagine a conventional cultural sequencing in which people prepare for work in their youth, become active full-time workers, and then fade gracefully into postwork life. All of these presumptions overstate experienced reality (Moen and Roehling 2005, 15; Pitt-Catsouphes 2005, 3). Members of Kristal's and Jeremy's cohort, and those who immediately follow them, must live within the restaging of adult experiences.

Full-time permanent work, especially in the kind of unstable high-technology and knowledge work of Silicon Valley, is problematic. Instead, people patch together an ecosystem of full-time employment, contract, or temporary work, and unpaid down time that reflects both the specific economy of the Valley and their families' needs. As we saw in the last chapter, the work strategies of the aging first wave required considerable reinvention. Once defined as the generation that followed the people born after World War II, Kristal's and Jeremy's cohort has come to be defined by the economic shifts have that hollowed out the American middle-class (Ortner 1998). People in this age cohort remain unconvinced that the conventional staging of prework, full-time work, and retirement will ever work for them. While flexible work scheduling was a radical invention to the older cohort, for those Jeremy's age and younger it has simply become the way work is done. Workers in this second wave cannot assume that their spouse, friends, or family will have the same work schedule that they do, or that their workplace will necessarily remain a stable source of income (Smola and Sutton 2002, 365). They are more willing than the first wave workers to rethink the personal consequences of work intensification (Benko and Weisberg 2007, 5). Must they settle for less personal satisfaction or the loss of family time?

Family sequencing is no more predictable than work sequencing. Couples may have children in their early twenties, or wait until their thirties, or even forties! A forty-year-old mother with young children may have more in common with another who gave birth at twenty-five than with someone her same age with teenagers or no children at all. Specific conditions matter more than age. High rates of divorce, widespread employment of middle-class women, and a fluctuating economy mean that workers who grew up in the last forty years do not expect a classic sit-com family in which men work and women stay at home.

While the second wave cohorts have been called "slackers," that stereotype reflects the angst of older journalists and pundits rather than the actual behavior of people born between 1961 and 1981. The pundits' anxieties about the larger economic changes of deregulation and employment instability became a moral panic about the death of the work ethic. The "pathologies of the world" were transferred onto that particular cohort (Ortner 1998, 419). Nonetheless, it is a legitimate observation that the subtle social contract that had governed employer-worker relations had changed from that offered to those born before 1960. Organizations and workers knew that economic flexibility might mean that workers, projects, divisions, and whole companies would be subject to elimination. Health and retirement benefits have eroded. Younger workers then chased higher salaries, all too aware of their own ephemeral status as they plot their course through diminished benefits (Smola and Sutton 2002, 365–78; Zemke, Raines, and Filipczak 2000, 124).

Especially in Silicon Valley, people in the second wave cohort spent their teenage years and early adulthood in a world dominated by digital devices. Mobile phones and Nintendo Wii game stations are part of their daily lives. In the United States, half of the workers aged twenty-nine to forty bank online. Like the first wave cohort, they use the Internet to search for health information. Eighty-four percent of second wavers use the Internet for health literacy (Fox 2005, 2–3). While they are not quite the gamers and instant messengers of those born in the late 1980s and the 1990s, this second wave cohort remain sophisticated users of social network and communications technologies. They can use this facility with online networking and mobile telephony to connect to friends, family, and acquaintances to collect and discuss specific practices for managing health—what to eat, how to move, and how to interpret medical mandates. They employ these behaviors themselves, and bring these experiments to spouses and children.

Adults from their late twenties to forty are at the age to establish families. These second wave workers are making the tricky transition from a person who is able to focus time and energy on work and play to one who must now accommodate a more complex landscape of responsibilities. Health becomes redefined not as a convenient source of individual productivity but as a moral value that is part of the social contract of adulthood. Taking care of someone else's health—partner, parent, child—is an ethical mandate. A new ecosystem of helpers has evolved to help these younger adults to navigate this set of responsibilities. This age cohort is composed of expert networkers who harness their social connections to help them take care of themselves and others. For the more elite, professional niches have appeared—life coaches, personal trainers, and therapists in company health facilities.

However helpful the network or organization may be, the onus for productivity and for embodied health remains the burden of the individual worker. Workers must discipline their emotions and bodies to work effectively and sustainably—in other words, to stay both healthy and productive. This internalized discipline has counterparts in other cultures. In this chapter, we will examine that discipline and compare it with its analogue in China, *suzhi*, the pervasive pursuit of personal quality. Yet Silicon Valley is not China, although many Chinese reside there. Fundamental cognitive schema, or orienting cultural frameworks, mold the way health and work are navigated in U.S. culture. People work on their own bodies to make them more productive, energetic, and focused. This discipline serves both the workers' self-interest and the interests of the larger economic system.

Amanda Stewart, Putting Transcendentalism in Place

In her day job Amanda is the director of a nonprofit organization, and her older husband works for a California state bureau. She comments, "Usually I have a lot of plants, because they're kind of healthy, give you good air. . . . I see health not just as my own physical fitness." She notes that now she is nearly forty, and so "I see . . . environment as a health issue. So we compost, we recycle, . . . I wish we had a grass yard that he could run around in." They don't have a lawn, so her son cannot run around, getting "aerobic exercise . . . but just getting out in the fresh air and the sun and the green, emotional health, the whole yard is good for that." We see an indication of a convergence of environmental thinking and health in Amanda Stewart's speculations about how she should reconstruct her Silicon Valley home now that she has a young son. Amanda remembers how she took vitamins, improved her diet, and lived more healthfully during her pregnancy, commenting, "I just wanted to give him the best chance at being healthy and strong."

Like that of her Transcendental forebears, Amanda's religious practice is eclectic, "cafeteria style. We have *The Way of Zen.* My husband has read a lot more about Zen and Taoism than I have." She comments that they live in the San Francisco Bay Area for a reason: more Chinese and Japanese Americans with a different perspective on "what health and wellness are." She notes that her husband, the household expert in things Asian, "was raised as a Catholic. I was raised as a Protestant and Presbyterian, but I'm not really either one. We're both more spiritual, more than we are religious. But being part of an environment and a community, being aware of yourself and at peace with yourself and doing good deeds, is what it's all about." Amanda points to her bookshelf; on it are "books related to spiritual things . . . that would be health related. More the wellness side . . ."

Transcendentalism, and its twenty-first-century incarnation in New Age beliefs, encompasses practices as diverse as natural healing, spiritualism, and technological optimism. These are not different models but different facets of a deeply imbedded American framework, one that took root especially in California and has a particularly obvious manifestation in the San Francisco Bay Area and Silicon Valley.

Silicon Valley's mixture of technological play and countercultural experimentation goes back to the nineteenth century, well beyond the iconic 1960s. Historically, Californians esteemed the region both as a "natural place" and as a site for nigh-utopian technocratic activity (Starr 2005, xiii).

People now living in that culture may have a difficult time articulating those values, but often merge these attitudes into an undefined optimism and "open-mindedness." Valuing nature, experimentation, and open-mindedness harkens back to the Transcendental movement in American cultural history.

In the historiography of American religious practice, intellectuals have usually categorized such experience as evangelical, metaphysical, or institutional—carrying on the traditions of the mainstream churches. Protestant evangelism is often seen as the central expression of American religious history. However, more recent analyses by historians Butler and Albanese suggest, not surprisingly, that the historic religious landscape was more complex. Immigrant and Native American folkloric traditions of magic and spiritualism merged with a new urban, middle-class "catholicity of mind and spirit, signified, especially, by an openness to Asia and an embrace of South and East Asian religious ideas and practices" (Albanese 2007, 2–12). By the mid-nineteenth century a distinctly American form of transcendental philosophy had emerged, which suggested that the natural abundance of the American environment made it a distinctly "noble" society—qualitatively different from other nations. The movement promoted a romantic cultural interpretation of world religion, emphasizing an individualistic spirituality and the belief in the inherent goodness of nature. Thoreau, one of the key proponents of this transcendent worldview commented, "The pure Walden water is mingled with the sacred water of the Ganges," reaffirming that connection to Eastern philosophies (ibid., 348). In the hybrid transcendental philosophy, nature is powerful, the mind is potent, and people are intimately connected to the environment and have a mandate to experiment on themselves (see Cramer 2004).

The manifestation of this "natural religion" in the lives everyday nineteenth-century Americans will seem familiar. If nature is good, healing with nature is best. From Sylvester Graham, of graham cracker fame, to Swedenborgian spiritualist missionary John Chapman, a.k.a. Johnny Appleseed, the linkage of discipline, spirituality, and nature was becoming firmly ingrained. Homeopaths, drawing on the emerging German medical system that used energy healing, and Naturopaths, who used traditional herbal approaches, competed with the early pioneers of biomedicine. In this transcendental worldview, the best practice would be to eat natural foods and vegetables, drink natural water, and that those nearest nature "would be in perfect health" (Albanese 1990, 122–23, 30).

Adherents were "preoccupied with mind and its powers," ranging from self-induced healing to technoscientific invention. They used the beliefs of naturalistic medical systems from India, China, and ancient Greece to consider correspondences—how the microscopic connects to the macroscopic. For example, a part of the body could be diagnostic of the whole person; the tongue or the eyes could be seen to be portals to the patient's state of being and health. Massage therapy in the ancient Hippocratic tradition forms the foundation for its revival in the late nineteenth and early twentieth centuries (Fuller 2005, 24–25).

Transcendental metaphysics holds that each person, in turn, reflects the larger society and environment, just as Chinese *feng shui* links the well-being of a person to the position of a home or workplace in the energetic landscape. Massage work on one part of the body is amplified to the whole person. Metaphysically, people and nature are composed of movement and energy, and that is more important than mere physicality (ibid., 375). Inherent in this worldview is "a yearning for salvation understood as solace, comfort, therapy and healing" (see Albanese 2007, 13).

Cultural borrowing is rampant in twentieth-century New Age holistic healing. These practices are the great-grandchildren of Transcendental healing; New Age philosophy connects inner emotional states and planetary health to personal well-being. Through time, disciplines as wide-ranging as chiropractic, osteopathy, yoga, Daoist healing, and *feng shui* have been fused into an aggregate and lumped into the ever-malleable New Age practices that had 10 million American adherents by the mid-nineties (ibid., 402–3, 509–11; see also English-Lueck 1990). The influx of Asian immigrants since 1965 intensified New Age interest in Asian practices (Albanese 2007, 484).

Contemporary transcendentalism is represented by New Age practices. Self-help actualization, and personal and societal transformation, are now mainstream ideas rather than deviations from American values. A study of New Age consumption in Texas demonstrated that the only real predictor of who would engage in "alternative" practices was whether someone in the person's network also practiced it. New Age consumption was spread across the demographic categories of age, ethnicity, class, education, and "conventional" religious practice (Mears and Ellison 2000). Another study, conducted out of Atlanta's MARIAL Center, on ritual, noted that among working mothers alternative medical practices spread through their families, media, or networks (LeVeen 2002, 6).

By the turn of the twenty-first century, 40 percent of U.S. adults had purchased complementary and alternative medical products (Eisenberg et al. 1998). In a study in 2002, a team from the National Institutes of Health found that 62 percent of the adult American population used complementary and alternative medicine (CAM) therapies, including prayer. Excluding prayer—although transcendental practices would warrant including it—36 percent of the population use natural products, do yoga or breath-related exercises, meditate, or use massage and chiropractic or diet-based therapies (Barnes et al. 2004, 1). Some 27 percent of all Americans use the Internet to search online for alternative health options, while 33 percent of Californians do so (Fox 2003, 12). In short, a significant portion of the American population engages in the use of alternative healing, enough to suggest it is no longer so alternative after all.

American Transcendentalism was a broad-ranging and free-spirited doctrine that valued experimentation. Novel approaches could be applied to natural conservation, astrology, and even engineering and health. The philosophy emphasized pragmatism and creativity, holding that the human mind is encumbered only by its own self-imposed limits (Albanese 2002, 21–24; Albanese 2007, 13). We see in John Muir (1838–1914) the embodiment of these cultural values (Albanese 2002, 11). He worked hard as a writer and political activist to preserve the wilderness in the United States, especially California's Sierra Nevada mountain range. He was also a naturalist and an engineer/inventor. Since his time, environmental activism has been linked to a romantic spiritualism that continues to view nature as reinvigorating. The invocation of **Gaia**, a consciousness attributed to the biosphere, is a natural outgrowth of transcendentalism (Albanese 2007, 508).

In the last chapter, we saw the first wave of cultural "revolutionaries" engage in social experimentation; they worked on transforming themselves. They brought together diverse cultural influences and wove them into a medically plural ecosystem of beliefs and practices. This older cohort reformed work organizations and the family itself to adapt to the emerging global knowledge economy. The second wave, slightly younger, also experiments on itself, fuses different cultures, and adapts to an economy that stresses individuation. For this cohort, however, the three processes of experimentation, cultural fusion, and adaptation are even less differentiated from each other and more tightly woven into everyday life.

Veeda Ferrazzi and Min Lee, Building an Ecosystem of Support

Veeda Ferrazzi, a native of the San Francisco Bay Area, is a forty-year-old mother of two young children and a researcher. Although frequent travel is part of her job, she can work from home and has created a space to do so. Veeda must also constantly produce to validate her virtual performance to colleagues and superiors who cannot monitor her directly. The work stress is intense. For a time she was falling prey to pathogens every time she traveled. She was constantly getting sinus infections and taking antibiotics. Then she began to reassess what was happening to her. Her husband, Roger, counseled her to nurture her body and let her immune system do the work. Veeda says, "It sounds really stupid, but I really could see the impact of sleep and rest. . . . So I started taking care of myself better, knowing that there was a real connection, for me at least. It was working for me."

She recognized that drinking water was a practice that she needed to integrate to keep healthy. Coffee dehydrates her, and wine, while part of living well, also dries her out. She was particularly careful while pregnant, but once she was back in her work routine the old habits started to re-emerge. She started drinking green tea. Veeda notes, "I start feeling dried out, my eyes burn. My nose is itchy because I'm dried out. So, drinking the tea—you put the water on and you boil it—reminds me to get hydrated."

Once she became aware of sleep and fluids, Veeda cultivated other practices to build her health. She chose the place she lives carefully, in order to be able to raise a healthy family. Veeda reflects, "We picked a place we knew was a walkable neighborhood, where we could get out every day and be outside—work in the garden or something—be close to public transportation." Both Veeda and Roger identify commuting as an emotionally and ecologically hazardous practice. She can do much of her project-based work independently on a computer, which gives her the flexibility to telecommute. Veeda also spends time in the new neighborhood with her intensely physically active sister, buffering the negative impact of sedentary work. Her moral commitment to her two daughters keeps her attention on developing a social and environmental infrastructure to keep herself, her family, and friends as healthy as possible. Veeda does not use extraordinary efforts to do so, but builds an ecosystem of incremental practices.

Veeda carefully manages the small details of her life, building in walks with her children and eating fresh vegetables from a local CSA (community supported agriculture) delivery service. Boxes of produce, whose contents vary with the season, are delivered to her doorstep. Exactly which fruits and vegetables she finds in the box is a surprise. Veeda remembers, "We got a flyer and said, 'Well, we'll try this one.' We were kind of ready to try it. That comes twice a month and it's great. You make do with what you get. So, I've learned how to do all sorts of things, things I never thought I would have cooked before. It's good! It's fun! There's all sorts of stuff. It's easy because *we're* not growing it. It is organic and that is something."

Veeda must also work face-to-face on teams and with clients, which forces her to make the long journey from Berkeley to Palo Alto. At her workplace, discussions of family and health create ties between people. Particularly in knowledge work and other team-based activities, where intangible thoughts are the medium of exchange, trust is a requisite element (Baba 1999, 333; English-Lueck 2002). While arguably the best way to build trust at work is to build a history of doing a job well, there are other tactics that people use to build trusting relationships. One way to build trust is to share details of life that create a sense of mutual vulnerability. Exchanging health-related information and stories about family build bridges between workers that facilitate trusting relationships. This strategy sweeps coworkers into the **personal health ecology** that family members need to find resources, disseminate knowledge, and make sense of complex and some-times contradictory health information. The stress experienced by juggling work and home can be turned on its head as coworkers become tacit family helpers. Veeda and her fellow workers share their own illness narratives and interventions, building intimacy. Similarly, family members become invis-ible and indirect coworkers, supporting intense bouts of productivity.

Veeda's health support system includes her sister, husband, and other kin, but also sweeps in coworkers and acquaintances. Her Silicon Valley workplace gives her obvious institutional support—supplying health care benefits and buffering her scheduling quandaries by providing flexible alternatives. It also provides distinct challenges, wearing her down and add-ing to her stress. Although it is far from her workplace, her neighborhood has tangible resources, such as places to walk safely. Veeda can contract for the delivery of organic produce from local farmers who routinely deliver to her neighborhood. She consciously cultivates this ecosystem of people, institutions, and practices, and in so doing, illustrates the strategies of sec-ond wave workers.

Min Lee illustrates this conscious cultivation as well, although she is in a position to command additional support from those under her control. Min is thirty, born in Seoul, South Korea. Recently diagnosed with diabe-tes, Min reflects that when she was growing up, even though her mother is fanatical about healthful food, she had been discouraged from participat-ing in sports because they were "unfeminine." She played varsity volleyball in high school, but her parents were uncomfortable watching her display herself quite so publicly. The eating habits she learned as a child are dif-ficult for her to change, especially cutting down on rice, a mainstay of an Asian family diet and an iconic symbol of Korean culture. Min tries, with mixed success, to enlist her family in her new eating and exercise strategies; it would be good for her mother, who also has diabetes.

Working in a stressful job with a frightening new diagnosis, she sees cre-ating a healthful workplace, one with less emotional strain and more physi-cal activity, as a priority. After her doctor, looking at her "dead-on," warned her that she must control her weight and her diabetes or risk potential birth defects for her unborn (and at this point only theoretical) child, she knew that she had to change her behavior. Min thought, "Oh my God, this is really serious. I've always been pretty conscious about preparing myself for when I do get pregnant. . . . I don't drink. I don't smoke. I've never done drugs. . . . Okay, I smoked pot once, but I didn't inhale! I've always been conscious about making sure I get my folic acid . . . preparing to have kids in the future. That's always been important to me." Min Lee has very specific reasons for changing her exercise and eating practices that are rooted not only in conventional disease management but also in her plans for child-bearing. Central to her motivation is preparing for parenthood, a moral imperative that appears again and again among young workers.

Min needed to create an ecosystem of support that extended beyond her family. Her solution was to use her position as a director to push for a "healthy workplace" and encourage her coworkers to exercise, relax, and take a healthful approach to work. After all, "I want them to take care of themselves and feel good about themselves, and I think you can only do that when you feel healthy." Her coworkers could then provide support for her to do the same. Alone she might not create these new, healthier practices. Her tactic was to use her position to redirect the goal of the workplace into supporting her efforts at health management. The worksite trainers and her nudged-into-being-supportive colleagues are now fixed in her health management ecosystem. Min uses a workout facility at her workplace, an on-site fitness center, but she has constructed a network of trainers and col-leagues to serve her health needs.

Veeda's support lies mainly in her family members and coworkers, occa-sionally drawing on institutions such as a farmer's cooperative. Min's nar-rative points to a larger ecosystem of specialists that help workers main-tain themselves efficiently. In addition to family members and coworkers, coaches, and trainers, personal assistants and therapists can be found in corporate workplaces, in gyms and spas, as practitioners or as independent consultants. The backgrounds of these specialists are as varied as their des-tinations. Some are alternative health practitioners, whose holistic healing credentials prepare them for spiritual, emotional, and embodied interven-tions. Psychology and business credentials can be combined to produce career coaches. Fitness experts—with backgrounds in kinesiology, physical therapy, nutrition, and sports—become credentialed as personal trainers. Others may draw on eclectic backgrounds to become personal assistants who manage the business of *life* for those who need to be totally dedicated to their work for the company. In a different culture and era the people performing many of these functions were called "servants." However, as bodies are remolded for productivity, the act of taking care of others is recast as *therapy*. Much of this therapeutic mandate is filtered through a transcendental lens, emphasizing individual agency, experimentation, and cross-cultural practices, and invoking a particular version of nature.

Jason, Margot, and Lily, in the Therapeutic Marketplace

Jason has assembled trainers into an independent fitness center, and he illustrates the concerns of those who supply the marketplace for self-improvement. Jason is forty, and his center caters to local companies, providing equipment, trainers, and other, less tangible services. He contacts companies and tells them of the flu shot clinics and blood drives that he runs as promotions. If you "serve the community . . . it comes back to you." Jason sits in his office, next to a calendar themed around disasters. One of his clients does failure analysis, and the calendar is a gift. His vitamins sit on his desk; he works long hours and does what he can to avoid getting sick. He goes out on the floor with his clientele, assessing their needs. In the beginning Jason provided a collection of industry magazines, but his clients wanted "an oasis for people to get away from work." So he now carries *Sports Illustrated*. He consciously steers conversations away from business, since his clients inevitably talk shop, by asking, "How about those Niners?" Ironically, he does not like sports, or support Oakland's football Raider Nation, but Jason keeps up with such news so that he can *talk* sports.

Jason's clientele is on the young end, averaging around twenty-eight, mostly male and drawn from an ethnically diverse population. There are tech stars in his clientele, founders of software companies and mentors in the industry, and there are "strong guys . . . but . . . mostly we have people that want to stay in shape . . . not body builders so much." He has been in the fitness business long enough that he sees a shift from a hard, steroid-using clientele to one much more attuned to health, people who "respect their bodies."

Margot occupies a very different niche in the ecosystem of services. She works directly on clients' bodies as a massage therapist. Margot received an associate of arts degree in massage therapy from a local community college, a "good program" but one completely based on anatomy and physiology. She injects her own brand of spirituality, drawing on the healing power of nature and communicating it to her clients. Margot draws her "energy from nature, however they want to interpret what nature is." Margot's business plan is simple; she contracts with the health provider of a major computer company, massaging clients at the tech campus itself. Her workspace is a quiet room with dimmed lights and scented oil—for those who are not allergic to the fragrance. She works with the health service nurse and ergonomicist, a person like Kristal. She refers carpal tunnel or other such problems to her colleagues. Margot's client pool, around 150 people, is mostly female. Many come to her directly, while others redeem gift certificates purchased by their managers as rewards for working "really long hours." Ironically, when project deadlines loom and her "people are so stressed," they are too involved with the work to come to her. During the most frantic phase of a project, when the workers really need relaxation, Margot rarely sees them.

Most of the time, Margot just massages their heads and shoulders. She likes to begin her massage at the feet, "because all these people are working with their head and that is where all the energy is. So I work at the feet first just doing some points. [I] just try to get some energy to come back down into the body." Later she moves her massage to the troublesome head and shoulders. Margot reflects, "I have clients who just lie there like a board, who have no concept that they have a body. They just have a head. Until their muscles are screaming at them, then they go, 'Oh yeah!'"

Lily provides a more indirect service, but one that is ultimately framed as therapeutic. Lily is a designer who has transformed her practice so that she composes interior landscapes according to the principles of *feng shui*. Lily distinguishes her practice from the faddish generic "diagram" approach and says, "I try to focus more on the classical approach which includes astrology.

It includes earth sciences, electromagnetic factors, and health factors. I also incorporate my business background into it." Her clientele "often times are very progressive, very in touch with New Age studies, which of course, isn't new. It's very old. It's . . . trying to bring these native, spiritual things back." She began learning years before from a Taiwanese professor who taught students at a local Buddhist temple. Some Americans, like Lily, went to Asia, learned the discipline, and brought it back. Lily notes that her practice has traction, not only among the region's Asian immigrants but also among the "culturally progressive" population of Northern California. Journalist Patricia Brown notes, "In California, *feng shui* is big business. In communities like Fremont and Cupertino, south of San Francisco, *feng shui* experts often consult with developers on the layout of subdivisions. . . . '*Feng shui* is a very major cultural factor,' said Irene Jhin, publisher of the *Chinese New Home Buyer's Guide*, based in Burlingame" (Brown 2004).

These "therapies," ranging from fitness training to spiritual interior design, are examples of the reach of the ever more complex health marketplace. In this book, most health and illness narratives are those of individual consumers of these practices, although they do create practices as well as consume them. Jason, Margot, and Lily provide a different perspective. The traditions and practices themselves, and those who provide them, have subtly changed. Exercise, massage, and *feng shui* have roots in antiquity, in Hippocratic medicine and traditional Chinese practices, but they are being organized through new institutional frameworks. Jason and Margot are allied with businesses in a subtle contract to keep workers supple. Realtors and local governments sweep in Chinese geomancy, using divination of earth energy, to accommodate both immigrant and transcendental beliefs. They are part of an ecosystem of therapeutic services that makes the transcendental disciplines of healthy living real, and even convenient.

Nikolas Rose, a social theorist who has applied Michel Foucault's notions of **governmentality** to bioscience and psychiatry, has identified several important themes in biomedicine that can be more broadly applied to the larger suite of practices constituting therapy, including alternative practices. Therapy has become a framework for reshaping "an individual's relations with others" and their "relationship with themselves." The advent of therapeutic governmentality provides a mechanism by which people "experience themselves and their world so that they understand and explain the meaning and nature of life-conduct in fundamentally new ways" (Miller and Rose 2008, 142–47). Therapy transforms the way we control ourselves and each other. Furthermore, the statistical revolution that produced biomedicine created a new objective for therapy, to achieve normalcy. However, the entry of "life enhancing powers of particular activities, foods, thoughts, and the like" shifts the goals of therapy from generic normalcy toward customization (Rose 2007, 20). Therapy is then directed toward the unique needs and desires of the client. The thrust of therapy is not simply bound "by the poles of health and illness," but directed toward "optimization" (ibid., 17). That optimization, or "self-actualization," is part of a discipline linked to entrepreneurism, maximizing an individual's capacity for innovation and agency (Miller and Rose 2008, 194).

The pool from which these therapeutic techniques are drawn is deeply diverse, blending nineteenth-century Transcendental concepts, expressions of a colonial global flow of ideas, and twentieth- and twenty-first-century exchanges of concepts, practices, and people. The production of bioscientific knowledge is global, but so are the discourses about alternative forms of therapy (see Photograph 6). In Silicon Valley, practitioners and clients are enacting globalized therapeutic disciplines.

In Silicon Valley, young adults have grown up with increasing cultural diversity, and while not necessarily "born to" deep diversity, they are active participants in encountering, engaging, and creating identities. Workers who have migrated to the Valley have done so to participate in the culture there; they are self-selected to place work as a central value in their lives and to embrace the deep diversity that allows the foreign-born and children of foreign-born to function there. In terms of health, this cultural cosmopolitanism translates into a comfort with medical pluralism. For example, while the widespread practice of yoga contributes to the medical diversity of the region, there is additional complexity below the surface. Northern Californian versions of yoga, practiced by the aging parents of these workers, exist side by side with the yoga practiced by the many varieties of Indian sojourners. Neelima Goti, a native of Bangalore, has a commercial yoga video, but her use of yoga and her blend of traditional Indian health practices are not the same as Amanda Stewart's, for whom a more American-adapted yoga simply helps her prepare for pregnancy. There is not one type of Ayurveda, the traditional health system of India, but many forms to choose from. These diverse practices range from an eclectic blending with biomedicine, often practiced by immigrants from India to versions that stress their distinction from biomedicine as practiced by Euro-American alternative healers. The core epistemology, American Transcendentalism, provides a foundation for integrating a host of beliefs that produce alternative health practices, an environment of experimentation and a work culture of invention. This collection of cultural values allows Silicon Valley workers, and many others, to turn their lives into experimental projects in deep medical diversity.

Addison Wu and Rupal Patel,
Locating Deep Medical Diversity

Addison Wu's problems are not unusual, and she illustrates some of the dilemmas facing young immigrants. Addison is thirty, lives with her parents, and works as a patient care coordinator at a dentist's office. Ethnically Chinese, Addison was born in Southeast Asia but has lived in Silicon Valley since she was two. Her parents wanted her to work in the computer industry, "because we do live in Silicon Valley!" Usually obedient, this time she said she would prefer to go into health care, although she decided against medical school because she disliked studying anatomy.

Addison is four feet, eleven inches tall, and now weighs a 105 pounds. As a teenager Addison was fit. In high school, she was subject to daily enforced physical activity, but that discipline dwindled when she went to college and began to work. Such activities become optional and therefore avoidable. College meant putting on that "freshman fifteen," and with her short stature, gaining weight is a problem. Addison reflects, "I was thin in high school, but after that, no sports, just munching. And that can get you really fat!" Her weight management had been effortless in high school, but the situation had changed. At 165 pounds she was warned by her doctor that "it was beginning to be dangerous." He scolded, "Be careful. You are still young, so be careful with it." It "started getting too much for me to handle, so I decided to do something about it and instead of going on diets, I decided I am maybe just going to eat smaller portions and exercise because I love to eat. Eating is part of my life. And if I can't eat what I want to eat that is bad. Bring on the fries! Bring on the ice cream!"

So Addison consciously decides to train to be fit. She began to exercise up to five times daily, aerobic workouts with her hula hoop, jumping rope, and body sculpting with weights—which she calls "her little buddies." Her stress level intensified when her grandmother died and she had to work more to get her sisters through college, as their tuition costs had shot up. She has to be careful of binge eating, saying, "I eat because the more I eat the less I think about my emotions. It was an emotional thing for me." Her "aunties" in Asia send her advice and remedies, such as Malaysian wheat grass, but she is content to focus on "eating dutifully" and exercise. She inserts workouts into every unused space in her life—at work, before and after dinner, in the middle of the night, sometimes sleeping only a few hours. She takes stairs instead of the elevator. She doesn't care for the large-scale gym infrastructure, preferring to use lightweight devices that she can use to monitor herself (see Photograph 7). She walks and tracks the calories used and steps taken with her mobile phone. For Addison, entering adulthood meant creating a training regime that matched her aging metabolism. Her workplace supports her new practices; she is allowed to use the waiting room for exercise when it is empty.

Addison, a young immigrant, illustrates some of the most obvious features of medical pluralism, as she joins together mainstream biomedical practices with Asian understandings and remedies. Her sphere of medical interaction, at least around her own care, is limited to her family and friends. Addison consults with her globally based kin and uses devices—designed for the individual—to help her watch and revise the program she has created for herself.

Rupal Patel's immigrant experience illustrates a different set of challenges. The American medical system remains a bit of a mystery to Rupal, although he understands the workaday world of high-technology well.

Rupal is thirty-one and has been in Silicon Valley for five years. The early years were simple. As an engineer from India, he submerged himself in the work with few distractions. Then his family arranged a marriage, and now he is a husband, the father of a one-month-old infant. Soon Rupal will host his diabetic mother for an extended visit to his small apartment in a gated apartment complex. He carefully manages his own health through diet and exercise, while working at least ten hours a day. The value of his workplace has subtly changed for him. No longer just a site of employment and professional development, his company provides the health insurance that seems essential now that he is a provider. Once a year he discusses his health plan with his company and reviews his coverage. His new family responsibilities bring higher premiums, but most of that is paid for by his employer.

In addition to dentists, doctors, and hospitals, Rupal says that he and his family often go to local Hindu temples as "part of our culture." Spiritual equilibrium is part of how his family members "maintain" their "health levels." For biomedical advice he can turn to his brother, who is a physician. They talk every day. If he doesn't feel good he waits for a time, trying to assess if there is really a medical issue. If the problem persists, he asks his brother, then his doctor, and then turns to the computer to do an Internet search.

Unfortunately, since moving to Silicon Valley and working for a large high-tech company, he has been gaining weight. Over at Google they call it the "Google twenty-five," similar to the "freshman fifteen"; these are pounds earned by a sedentary lifestyle. Gourmet cafeteria food is just too tempting. After his marriage Rupal realized that he now had responsibilities, and keeping his health in order was part of that moral mandate. So Rupal talked to his brother, searched the Internet, and structured a diet plan. He got a personal trainer and started going to the gym. He has had his body finely tuned—to be fit and productive.

Then the baby was born. He can't tell whether his child is normal or unhealthy—the whole experience is too "new." He talks to his friends and his daughter's doctors and puzzles his way through parenting. His wife is on maternity leave and he helps, saying, "As a father, I do my stuff." Rupal also monitors his mother's health. She has diabetes, and every week her numbers must be assessed. While she talks to her doctor, Rupal scans the web for information. He finds foot creams, and reads about her medications. He discovers a new world of devices and services that he relays to his mother. The responsibilities are beginning to mount. He looks into the future and realizes that forty is not so far away after all, and "we will have to be very careful."

Generally positive about his adult responsibilities in his home and workplace, he is less sanguine about the American medical system. Having to wait a month to get an appointment seems ludicrous; in India he would just walk into the office of the doctor of his choice and be seen. Why should he end up with a total stranger? He finds it hard to elicit information from the doctor. He doesn't just want to have instructions about what to do; he wants to understand why the illness is happening. He dislikes having to find a pharmacist to query. Shouldn't the doctor be explaining potential side effects and interactions? Rupal wants a thorough explanation. After all, he *is* an educated man. He admires the technology of the medical system of the United States but not the delivery system itself. Rupal functions well within multiple medical beliefs but has trouble with the system that delivers care that potentially interferes with his ability to be a responsible husband, son, and father.

Both Addison and Rupal draw on a global set of traditions for specific practices and beliefs; even the majority of their activities that could be identified as health-related stem from biomedicine. They have woven together biomedical notions and practices from their distant relatives. However, the imperative of second wave workers remains intact. They must work on themselves, to correct potential problems and to stay fit. That particular agenda, to stay fit, is intertwined with familial obligations and habits of thinking from their respective professions in health care and technoscience.

Luke Brandeis, Staying Well and Better than Well

Practicing complementary and alternative care, as Luke does, adds another dimension to medically diverse self-experimentation. Luke Brandeis embraces a variety of devices and practices just to manage his chronic conditions and uses them to augment his day-to-day functioning.

A thirty-nine-year-old intellectual, Luke has Type 1 diabetes, poor vision, and **Marfan's syndrome**, a genetic condition that has resulted in a damaged heart valve. He received an artificial heart valve at eighteen. Luke explains: Marfan's syndrome is "a condition of the ligaments and joints, and Abraham Lincoln had it. In general it makes you tall and it makes your joints elongated. Unfortunately, though, it also expands your aortic heart valve. . . . I was eighteen, and I felt like my back stiffened up when I was on the way back home from school, and apparently the valve was expanding, so they had to replace it." When he is quiet, you can hear it beat. He uses his glucometer five or ten times a day to monitor his glucose and charts it on his computer. Luke is adding an insulin pump to the technologies that keep him alive. As his support system grows, Luke meditates on what this means to him:

> It comes back to where do *you* as an individual end and your body begin? That was becoming really blurry with me. The same thing goes back to feeling dependent on devices. Now I have a device implanted within me that I utterly depend on its functioning to work . . . a second device. So I feel like I'm in this web of devices—devices that I have to carry with me, devices that may be part of me, devices that are already inside of me. I'm always for whatever works, right up to stem cell research, and animal research too. . . . So the cyborg thing, I think I had that even at age twelve. I was thinking, "Oh, I'm dependent on this device now. This device is a real extension of me now. . . . The only thing it doesn't give me is superpowers." And I'm like, damn, you know. What it does give me is an extra sense of my body though. . . . It gives me that feeling of power that I think not everyone has. So in that sense, it's a psychic shift really.

Yet Luke has many tools at his disposal to enhance his life, in addition to the medical devices that sustain it. The advent of low-carbohydrate diets has made new products available to him, from Diet Coke to high-fiber power bars. "It's like a diabetes paradise." Luke's brother is "into Tony Robbins," an entrepreneur who has capitalized on neurolinguistic programming-style self-help seminars. Anthony Robbins has created a global coaching empire. He sells products and seminars, designed as self-actualization tools, to guide people to live an "extraordinary life." Luke's house is decorated with Tony Robbins affirmations that he uses to fine tune his attitude: "You can do it!" "Eat well." "Today is the time for exercise," "This is the place to be." He is sensitive to the power of words.

Place also matters to Luke. He is conscious of place and knows the value of each spot: particular places to meditate, the neighborhood streets where he walks, and the grocery stores that carry the products he can eat. He tests his blood in specific locations, where he also goes to meditate on his life. In the main hallway he has a spot where he tests after he comes back from his morning constitutional. He has other places in his home as well, "like a medical workstation . . . a meditation area too. It's a place where I can check in with my body." Luke takes a "poll" of his body, tracking whether his blood sugar is in range, but also looking at the bigger picture. He meditates on, "Am I doing okay? What could I be doing better? Do I need to do more exercise? Do I need to eat less? I can always check in to see what my body chemistry is, and I love that."

Luke's in-laws work for Whole Foods and have influenced his wife to explore the holistic approach of Andrew Weil—a leader in integrative medicine from the University of Arizona. Luke began to experiment with adding new practices, especially around food, and rethinking his health management. He says, "It just got me more mindful. I think it was that development of mindfulness of health that was really important . . . really thinking about the mind/body connection . . . again, checking in with my body made me feel better about myself." Beyond the consciousness his "cyborg" status gave him, he "re-evaluated the way I was testing my blood . . . thinking that there were different ways to approach medicine than from a Western point of view." He began to practice meditation and does yoga and *taiji*. He visits acupuncturists and yet is still perfectly comfortable at his **health maintenance organization**. Luke is, after all, "an HMO baby." He divides his life into the cyborg phase, the holistic phase, and then wonders, "What's next? It's like, now I'm ready for the cure. I'm ready for the genetic phase where they just cure it!" Luke is not just maintaining his health, but using global alternative remedies, organic food, and nutraceutical food supplements to augment it. For Luke, the world of transhuman augmentation—being better than well—blends seamlessly into the medically plural realm of transcendental natural healing.

Luke's practices hint at more than simply *staying* well, but being *better than well*. There is a subtle distinction. Being healthy is part of an older discipline of self, one that suggests maintenance and repair. To be *augmented* is to be improved, through health practices or technologies, making a person "transhuman." A highly debated philosophical term, "transhumanism" is an "intellectual and cultural movement that affirms the possibility and desirability of fundamentally improving the human condition through applied reason, especially by developing and making widely available technologies to eliminate aging and to greatly enhance human intellectual, physical, and psychological capacities" (Bostrom 2008).

In Silicon Valley, transhumanism takes on many forms: including active meet-up groups that identify with the movement and those who simply accept the notion that augmentation is an appropriate metaphor for humanity. Silicon Valley's role in promoting the concept of augmentation is deeply rooted in its development. Early in the development of computing, the dominant model for technological development was *replacement*, aiming toward functional artificial intelligence. Computing pioneers such as Doug Engelbart posited a new direction, using technology to *augment* human intelligence (Markoff 2006, 45–47, 66–67). Before such substances earned notorious reputations, in the early 1960s, experiments with LSD sensitized Bay Area intellectuals to the notion of cognitive augmentation. Some participants in these psychological experiments founded the computer science Augmentation Research Center, where the ideas behind the mouse, the typewriter-derived QWERTY keyboard, and the CRT terminal were developed (Turner 2006, 61, 107–8). Technology would augment human intelligence, helping people produce, communicate, and *be* more efficient. The metaphor of augmentation changed the way technology was conceived, invented, designed, and implemented.

In a tone reminiscent of Addison, feminist sociologist Gimlin's ethnographic study of an aerobics class in New York revealed that the women have a nostalgic memory of their bodies, and talk about having somehow "lost" their ideal bodies. They turn to exercise and, as they age, sometimes cosmetic surgical intervention (Gimlin 2002). Such interventions are well used in Silicon Valley by those who can afford them. Appearance, as Giddens notes, is part of the project of self-actualization (1991). In a culture that celebrates youthful innovation, appearing aged or looking tired is a liability. Dr. Cheng, a Los Gatos cosmetic surgeon, comments that his patients prefer incremental changes to radical ones. Starting in their thirties and forties, they want to "keep what they have." They also do not want to lose work time. He comments, "In Silicon Valley in particular, people want quick fixes with little to no downtime because they're too busy to wait out a long healing process." So they pursue the small corrections of collagen tissue fillers and blepharoplasty to de-puff lower eyelids. Older clients opt for more expensive and consequential augmentation. Another surgeon, Dr. Weston, comments that more people, women and men, are trying to "stay vital in a precarious workplace. ... There is a premium placed on youth here" (Kato 2004). Cosmetic practices that are used to pursue the appearance of vitality become augmentation.

Cosmetic surgery, once a technology of repair, has become something to enhance existing experience. In a similar way, medical technologies originally designed to treat cognitive and affective disorders are expanding to augment attention, memory, and learning in healthy people. The field of **cosmetic neurology** is beginning to emerge (Chatterjee 2007, 130–31), as people begin to tinker with their neurochemical selves (Miller and Rose 2008, 104–5). There is a whole suite of prescription medications to help people focus or be more productive in school or work. Often in pill form, nutraceuticals—food or herb derivatives that are marketed to have an impact on human health—range from well-known vitamins to specific plant or animal derivatives. Well-made "gourmet" coffee, such as that favored by Veeda, Kristal, and Jeremy, provides a caffeine boost. In the words of Paul Erdős, "A mathematician is a machine for turning coffee into theorems" (Reid 2005, 16). Kristal's Mango·Xan is an example of an "energy inducing drink" that is also supposed to be able to reduce inflammations. **Functional foods**, which provide a health benefit beyond nutrition, are also examples of augmented nutrition. Examples range from breakfast cereals with oats to enhance heart health to organic eggs with omega-3, produced by feeding flaxseed to hens (see Nestle 2002, 333–34). Dairies add vitamin D to milk, and Coca Cola adds vitamins to its Diet Coke Plus. People in this younger second wave cohort are comfortable with these functional foods (Belasco 2006, 251).

Janelle and David Smith, Adult Onset

The second wave cohort, whether they are just beginning career and family at twenty-five or forty, is coming into the full impact of adult responsibilities. Young parents and parents-to-be, such as Luke, Rupal, Jeremy, and Kristal, consciously prepare themselves for their new duties. Self-care becomes family-care, an inherently moral endeavor. The family occupies a special position in the American social structure. It is the site of accommodation for other institutions. The family is the visible arena "where problems are expressed, even if causes lie elsewhere" (Darrah 2005, 12). The family home is the first and last bastion of health care. Symptoms are felt by family members, and their kin help them understand whether an embodied feeling is an illness or simply one of the normal miseries of life. Heath care decisions are based on the resources collectively harnessed in the home from employer-based insurance or network-based expertise. Religiosity and cultural values are embedded, disseminated, and debated within the confines of the family. The busyness of life, referenced earlier—managing the many activities that fall to an individual worker, student, patient—is navigated within the family. That navigation means making particular decisions within an ecosystem of choices, many of which are constrained or benefited by specific work circumstances.

Parenting becomes the navigation of risk, trading one potential danger for another in the moral quest to take care of the next generation (Beck 1992, 22–27). Risk, as Rose points out, is a function of thinking and acting after potential futures have been considered (2007, 70). Public health discourses have been the medium through which health risks for families and workers have been translated. There is a long-standing structural connection between work and family through modern public health strategies. In the nineteenth century, from sewer gas to germs, the home was seen as a place of lurking dangers. Food was distributed in the home. Sanitation in the home—private hygiene—was seen as an essential element of public health. Cleaning the home was the domain of women in the cult of domesticity; it was also a critical health practice and gave rise to a whole industry (Tomes 1997, 506–7). In the twenty-first century, the linkage between hygiene and moral parenting is less oriented toward pathogens, although that connection is still there. Rather, families now struggle to protect themselves from pollutants, toxins, and environmental degradation (ibid., 521).

The tension between work and family in U.S. culture is so poignant precisely because both are such powerful centers of moral action. Being a good parent means expending considerable effort to take care of the well-being of the next generation. That may mean making sure that the children are educated and prepared for the workforce, and that they haven't been unduly exposed to industrial toxins in their school or agricultural toxins in their food. Moral action in the family can be manifest in making breakfast, or in taking civic action to monitor **superfund sites**. Workplaces can be allies in this pursuit through "family-friendly" and "wellness" policies, and certainly coworkers can be confederates in making family life satisfactory. However, both workplaces and colleagues can also be barriers to health as well, by emphasizing the morality inherent in the work ethic at the expense of the workers and their families. Devotion to work is a central tenant of the productivity ethic, and not to be easily set aside.

Janelle and David Smith both work in education. They embody the complexity of juggling dual knowledge service-based careers and a young middle-class family. They also illustrate the diverse cultural alternatives from which they must consciously choose. As parents and educators, they must make decisions that reach beyond themselves to influence the next generation. Experimental, deeply diverse, and intensely productive, Janelle and David model the challenges faced by their age cohort. Janelle is a speech pathologist; her family is from Panama, and she bilingual in Spanish. David Smith is a residence director (RD) at a Silicon Valley University, a young African-American professional with jurisdiction over "student life" on campus. Because of his work, they reside on campus in a tiny two-bedroom apartment inside a residence hall, the only young family in a sea of eighteen-year-olds. Mirella Smith is only a few weeks old. Her older sister, Mardi, is not yet three. They carefully planned both Mardi's and Mirella's births to fall during academic breaks. Mirella has her mother for an eight-week maternity leave, including the Christmas holiday, before Janelle returns to her rounds in San Jose's elementary schools. Mardi is thoroughly integrated into her parents' working lives. Another RD, Toni, has been adopted as an "auntie" and helps them with the logistics of their "revolving door" childcare strategy. One parent goes to work as the other returns. They meet for breakfast, hand off the children, then meet for dinner and switch. This particular weekend David is on a twenty-four hour shift, on-call at any time of day for crises that can range from quarreling roommates to serious infringements of university regulations. He is particularly good with "judicial" issues, knowing when to transform the infringement into a life lesson, and when to deem it a legal matter for the campus police. It's the end of the holidays, and they have returning students and visiting relatives from the Midwest, all wanting to see the new baby. David gets up first, his PDA beeping to remind him to pick up the cloth diapers that have been delivered. He checks the digital monitor that allows him to hear what is going on in his daughters' room, although the apartment is small enough that such electronic eavesdropping is a bit redundant.

Janelle wakes next and talks to David about buying groceries; she wants the ingredients for Panamanian rice—peas, coconut oil, and *bakala* as well, a salty dried cod fish. Her mom pipes up that she didn't take the train from the Midwest to cook for them. David mentions that he is an excellent cook and makes a mean stir-fry. Janelle playfully asks him if he wants a stir-fry cookoff, but he says he would need a wok. Janelle scoffs, "You don't need a wok. You're not the iron chef!" Ultimately they settle on red snapper. They have a tiny kitchen, and it bursts with cooking supplies. They also have the option of eating in the dining commons with the residential students, which they do when work ramps up and they struggle to find the time and energy to cook and clean.

Exercise becomes another casualty of working parenthood. David, a near-professional basketball player, continues to practice through injury and distraction. His games can be family events. Janelle, however, finds it hard to make time for her own exercise. Walking strollers is not the same workout as rollerblading with age-mates. Televised *Tae Bo* is hard to do in a one-meter-square space in a cramped apartment.

While Janelle and Mardi are playing, David goes into his office and prepares an event for the hall, related to a couple of cases of substance abuse in the previous year. Roofies, Roche's Rohypnot, the insomnia treatment turned "date rape drug," and Ecstasy, methylenedioxymethamphetamine (MDMA), "the rave drug," are intimated. He plans to do some serious education on substance abuse before student infractions become real criminal activities.

A few weeks later, the temporary reprieve of parental leave draws to a close. The whole family goes to the doctor for Mirella's well-baby visit. They are covered by Blue Shield, but this visit is a no-co-payment, long wait sojourn. They settle in the pediatrician's office. Janelle picks up a *Working Woman* magazine, to see if her career remains among the twenty hottest. When Mirella gets fussy, Janelle walks her around, greeting the other babies happily until another mother comes in with her sick nine-month-old. He has had the flu since Monday and she has to work. The mother wonders, "Why isn't he getting better?" Her husband and she both work, and she needs this taken care of before the weekend. Her family is in Mexico and Nebraska, and her sister didn't come to help until a couple of months ago. She tells Janelle that she doesn't think she will have another; she just did not realize how time consuming babies could be.

Mirella's well-baby check goes mostly well; she is gaining an appropriate amount of weight and is thriving on breast milk, "the good stuff." She does have an umbilical hernia that may resolve in the next few months. David is a little concerned, especially when the word "surgery" is used. Shot time. The range of required vaccinations is available in only three shots, which are done deftly. As long as Janelle holds her, Mirella is fine.

As the next year unfolds, the Smiths discover what Janelle had already experienced, as a speech pathologist, that "all life revolves around sick kids." Mardi is generally healthy but has "poop issues." She is chronically constipated, with discomfort and medical response escalating over the course of five months. It takes a year to find the right specialist and begin to address the underlying causes, a year that takes a toll on the whole family (see Darrah, Freeman, and English-Lueck 2007, 61–62). Janelle and David are juggling working across several sites and accommodating complex work-related social demands. A sick child "speeds up the treadmill of quality parenting" and requires that much more effort (Jarvis and Pratt 2006, 338).

The Smiths form a dual-career family, one that illustrates that children are part of an ecosystem that includes adult work, food choices, exercise patterns, identity play, and attitudes toward life. Mirella and Mardi are reflective of their own identities, learning Spanish, playing with multicultural sticker books. When Mardi gets eighteen Barbie dolls for her birthday from family, friends, and parents' coworkers, the majority of them are "African-American," embodying a particular cultural identity. Children are socialized into this world, but also act as anchors for parental agency. Children are transformed by their parents and revolutionize the options of those around them, opening some windows for reflective self-conscious work and health management among the adults, and closing others. Parental health attitudes and behaviors define the routines that shape children's health practices (Tinsley 1992, 1046–48).

Debate on the navigation of work and family life can be framed in many ways. Workplaces and families can be seen as organizational units. The impact of the interaction of work and family can be analyzed through its individual workers and family members. However, recalling that both work and family are embodied processes recasts the discussion of their interaction. Both work and family life are being redesigned for productivity. People struggle to make their bodies well, or even better than well, to serve the adult obligations of family and work.

Policies meant to "improve" work and family balance can themselves have unanticipated implications if "bodies" are left out of the program. In her study of lactation-friendly workplaces in the Bay Area, sociologist Bentovim notes that women curiously ignore the reality of bodies in the workplace. Nursing mothers are expected to **breast pump** milk in seclusion—yet another task to be worked into a hectic day. The real business of lactation is messy—breasts leak—and requires a relaxation hard to achieve in the corporate ladies' room. Bentovim found that women developed strategies and stories to maximize their productivity both in making milk and reaching project milestones. Women pumped while multitasking, reading email, or in the car. Breast-feeding became another project to be managed. Leslie, a self-employed consultant, noted, "In my mind, the distance from Fremont to Mountain View is three ounces" (Bentovim 2002, 10–12).

Janelle Smith, a speech pathologist, owned a pump, but her infant daughter, Mirella, was "truly offended by the bottle." Janelle then had to create tiny windows of opportunity to feed Mirella. She could quickly drive home after the end of her school day, nurse Mirella, and then quickly return to conduct meetings with teachers and parents about her speech pathology clients. If Mirella did not wake up during that critical window, the remainder of the day's routine would be in jeopardy. Mothers are fully aware that nursing is an embodied experience; employers, even those who are "lactation-friendly," treat workers as ideally disembodied. Working mothers have to accommodate the assumptions that steal away their bodies. While devotion to the family is clearly a moral mandate, so is commitment to work.

Working on Bodies, Working on Self

The larger infrastructure of employer-based health care is being transformed. The pool on which risk is assessed is becoming more and more fragmented, making it difficult to keep costs down for the employers who contribute to worker benefits. Premiums to third-party payers are skyrocketing, and the relative contribution of the employee is increasing. Even the category *employee* is problematic, as expert and unskilled labor alike become contingent workers, differing from direct employees entitled to health benefits (Barley and Kunda 2004). We will explore this situation in more detail in Chapter 5, but the consequences of this change are clear—a greater burden for individual workers and their families, as they must work harder and longer to meet their responsibilities. Employers are caught in the middle, trying to keep benefits that traditionally helped retain workers, offering new services that help their employees stay healthy, while still maintaining their bottom line.

Workplaces like Cisco are experimenting with a new model of care, de-emphasizing sick care, which is the most expensive, and augmenting preventative wellness programs. Wellness programs are notoriously difficult to manage, and long-term benefits to individual companies are difficult to defend when there is high employee turnover (Galvin and Delbanco 2006, 1550). Nonetheless, particularly when employees are "high value," there is sufficient motivation for corporate experimentation. For example, in Cisco's pilot program employees are given a cash incentive to participate in health risk assessments, and additional rewards for behaviorally implementing health advice. Workers with health problems are given coaching to help them understand and materialize behavioral changes that should reduce the chance of developing expensive advanced chronic conditions. By 2007 more than half of the employees had taken such assessments, and 65 percent of those eligible for coaching were using the service (Moos 2007).

Essential to this wellness approach is the use of a broad definition of health, such as the World Health Organization's assessment of a healthy workforce as one that is healthy, productive, ready, and resilient (Hymel 2006a, S6). Employee-based wellness programs are part of a larger ecosystem of changes designed to reduce health care cost by increasing efficiency. Some of those changes are directed at employees' lifestyles and personal habits. Such a broad definition penetrates the daily lives of workers, going well beyond workplace concerns into the family and community. In principal, American workers support such efforts, although they are more skeptical of wellness programs in their own particular workplaces when their personal privacy is at stake (Helman, Greenwald, and Fronstein 2007, 4–5). Implicit in this organizational experiment is the necessity that the workers take on a new project for their company—themselves. Employees must compete for organizational resources, guard against stress, and work to prevent chronic illness; at the same time they must demonstrate their dedication to job productivity.

The competitive self-management and the tactical promotion of health practices converge to create a **health ethic** that harnesses the discipline of the work ethic and applies it to the crafting of self. This convergence of values and practices is similar to those actions that swirl around narratives of the word *suzhi* in the People's Republic of China. Increasingly, over the past few decades, Chinese citizens are described as having low or high *suzhi*—that is, as people of poor or good quality.

Over the last fifteen years, sinologists have been increasingly fascinated by the way the government, the media, and everyday folk in China talk about *suzhi*. Most frequently translated as "quality," *suzhi* is an expression whose meaning is morphing, expanding, and being adapted. The use of this concept by the Chinese state became associated with Deng Xiaoping's market socialism. For this reason, most of the analyses of the term are overtly Foucauldian, relating the discipline of everyday behavior to the power of governmentality (see Murphy 2004; Yan 2003; Anagnost 2004). High quality was explicitly associated with being educated, urban, cosmopolitan, innovative, and competent in the market. Just as the "socialist man" embodied characteristics desired by the Chinese Communist Party generations before, the new citizen-consumer supported a vision of a wealth-generating and thoroughly modern China. Those who enacted these values had a high level of *suzhi*, to be contrasted with rural peasants whose attachment to folk religion, clan consciousness, and gambling marked them as having low *suzhi* (Yan 2003, 498). *Suzhi* would be "taught and tested" in the educational system, tacitly marking separate tracks for the menial and mental workers of the future. A well-educated urban innovator with only one child who has a strong, but not strident, nationalism has profoundly high *suzhi*. Since the term emphasizes individual quality by validating a "personal moral code," it could shift the burden of responsibility for productivity, education, family management, and even health to the individual and away from the government (ibid., 510). Does this shifting of responsibility sound familiar?

Yet the Chinese government, despite its one-party system, is not a uniform entity, and messages coming from one bureau in Beijing may differ from the understanding of another, or of a municipality. It is not a simple matter of governmental hegemony. Moreover, now that the term is in the popular imagination, it can be applied to a wide variety of circumstances to mean a variety of desirable characteristics. The term *suzhi* can signify many different things, and individuals can play with the definition to position themselves favorably. Urban teenagers use *suzhi* to denigrate rural or ethnic migrants. Otherwise top students who test poorly can be painted as having poor psychological *suzhi*. Students who test well can claim *suzhi* by study-ing assiduously, showing that they have developed inner discipline (Fong 2007).

Embodied disciplines include not only studying and urbanity but also well-being. Medical anthropologist Judith Farquhar has done decades of research on the role of Chinese medicine in everyday life. Food, pleasure, and medicine converge to create the Chinese version of the "good life" (Farquhar 2002; see Farquhar 2007). As she wryly notes, all food is politi-cal, embedded in notions of nationalism, farm policy, and of course, *suzhi* discourses. Along with Zhang Qicheng, Farquhar closely examines *yang-sheng*, "life-cultivation arts," in Beijing, which promote health, well-being, and *suzhi*. *Taijiquan* and *Qigong* are classical examples of such individual practices, but so are photography, dancing, or taking walks to "soak up the sunshine and air, that is, in theory, fresh" (Farquhar and Zhang 2005, 306). With the dismantling of socialist health care access, Chinese citizens increasing "realize that they are on their own" (ibid., 319–20). Building their quality through life-cultivation arts is an adaptation to this reality. *Suzhi* is a deeply malleable qualifier with no English counterpart, yet it helps us understand how culturally shaped internal discipline can embrace a range of domains, from improving health to redefining work practice.

Specific moral actors—daughters, sons, parents, coworkers, physicians—are the agents of this discipline. The word *discipline* conjures up an image of social theorist Michel Foucault. He suggested that diffuse, pervasive, but passive conventions—nonagentic power—shape the discourses and actions of people. An anthropologist might call those ambiguous tropes "culture," or point out that the beliefs can bind individuals fast into structures of power. The work ethic, for example, deeply benefits the generic structures of capitalism by intensifying productivity. The work ethic encourages disci-plines that profit industry. A health ethic shapes the morality of consump-tion—of health products or services—which also benefits productivity (see Miller and Rose 2008, 116). Tracking that embodied "socially constituted agent" of discipline through specific situations can tell us how power is navigated and experienced (see Sangren 1995, 5–13). For the embodied workers of Silicon Valley, it is useful to ask: who are the agents of discipline, how do they rationalize their actions, and what factors enhance and constrain this "ethic"? The actual experience of disciplining oneself may serve the structures of power and at the same time create alternatives to subvert that power.

Rachel Cohen, Getting a Game Face

Rachel is a journalist, and she reflects on how important it has been to be conscious of how her embodied emotions will be read. When she was growing up, in Berkeley, she thought she was "not a terribly complicated person." She cried when she was sad and laughed when she was happy. She had observed that "there are people in the world [for whom] those equations aren't necessarily true." When she went into the working world she realized, "It's usually pretty easy to read what's going on in my face. A friend of mine from work once said, 'You don't have a game face. You need to get a game face.'" She thought about whether that discipline applied to her and concluded it did not. She lived in a truly diverse place, where people "are not like you," and while it might be useful to have such discipline, it would also be problematic.

Rachel, while she works with ideas and people, does not work in a high-tech environment. There, a different ethic may prevail. Sharone and Melton, in their various ethnographies of high-tech workplaces, emphasize the requirement of "competitive self-management." Individuals engaged in project work must manage themselves so that they make their companies competitive. They are also rivals to others in their own project team, and those on other projects within their companies. Individual workers must compete as well as cooperate. Hence while engineers may work long hours, because that "is up to the individual," they are making that choice within a context of competitive self-management (Sharone 2002, 1–6). Performance metrics reinforce this competition. Getting a 3.5 score on a performance review means that doing better than average really is just keeping up with the pack (ibid., 12). Self-selected high achievers are catapulted into a competitive self-management spiral as high goals are reset to even higher ones. These workplaces set a culture of "time-demands" that value working long hours and reward the virtuous who are willing to meet them (Mennino, Falter, Rubin, and Brayfield 2007, 488).

Along with this pervasive and intense sense of competition comes a form of emotional self-management quite different from Rachel's. **Emotion work,** especially in science and technology work, is an important mechanism for communicating rationality and control. In project teamwork optimism and enthusiasm are rewarded, but anger, fear, and frustration are not. These embodied moderations are learned in engineering schools, and favor those who tone down their emotional expression. For those who are not comfortable with such introversion, particularly women, this is a challenge (Melton 2003, 104–7). People learn when to keep their "game faces" and when to groan and make faces in frustration—inside the safety of a cubicle or with trusted coworkers. However, expressing frustration about too much work, tales of overwork, is allowable. Such grousing reveals that a person is working hard, and that sentiment reinforces that work is serious business (ibid., 110).

Aaron, a software engineer, says that his workgroup has a "Timex award" given to the person who has generated the most stress-related illnesses. That person can "take a licking but keep on ticking" (English-Lueck 2002, 68). This ritual demonstrates, with irony, dedication to the ethic of competitive discipline. This phenomenon is particularly acute in technology rich workplaces where time is "compressed and accelerated," and information overload is accompanied by heightened pace of work. Financial journalist Jill Andresky Fraser (2007, 143–44) calls this experience "technostress." The intangibility of knowledge work makes being *seen working* all that more important. One aspect of the need to be seen working can be measured in the unintended consequence of "presenteeism," dragging oneself to work even when ill, fearing the social and economic consequences of being absent (Middaugh 2006, 103–5).

Manipulating and enhancing one's body in the service of productivity is a moral act. The individuation of work—in which workers have become more responsible for their own productivity—is clearly one force that influences workers' lives. It is not the only moral force in play. Work is valued, given primacy, and embodies an ethic of mastery and discipline. Yet, when the burden of productivity is given to the individual, there is a potential for that ethic to sweep in all aspects of life into the service of work. What are the moral safeguards for preventing that restructuring of life?

Here again, health is important. As people are enhancing themselves to be better than well, and forcing ill bodies to continue to produce, health may still be invoked to buffer the demands of work. Even in Silicon Valley, our social conventions consider illness to be a mitigating circumstance for continued productivity. We do have "sick days" as a cultural category that can be called upon to manage the demands of work. Veeda's continued sinus infections and Min's diabetes allowed them to push back on work's demands by using a competing virtue. In that formula, health is a collective, not an individual, enterprise, and to abandon sick coworkers to their fate is an immoral act. There are socially defined moral limits of what can be asked of unhealthy people. Illness is a clear refuge against the demands of work intensification, as well as a probable consequence. People have agency in recognizing and invoking the collective moral stance to protect the ill and to buffer themselves from what they consider to be unreasonable demands.

Although Silicon Valley has no specific word for it, such as *suzhi*, there is a comparable disciplining of self. Disciplining the body is intimately linked to self-actualization, making *self* a project that embraces "appearance, demeanor, sensuality" and "regimes" (Giddens 1991, 99). Part of that discipline is what is commonly identified as a work ethic, a value set that is alive and well in a region whose main purpose is work. Few people come to Silicon Valley just to enjoy the climate and scenery. Another facet of that discipline is emotional control, which is linked to the self-discipline of teamwork and work in a multicultural setting. Working in deep diversity requires the emotional control to refrain from reacting to inadvertent cultural faux pas (English-Lueck 2002, 131–33). While education is valued, particularly by immigrants, creativity is the intellectual attribute most celebrated in local discourse. Creativity is the key to innovation, which is the raison d'être of the region. Finally, organizations are shifting to employee wellness programs, focusing on behavior as the root of chronic disease. This innovation merges training for health into other work disciplines. In order to be a "good worker," the scope of life to be managed broadens to include health management. As Valerie O'Hara writes in her self-help book on wellness in the workplace, "[T]he key to wellness is your own firm resolve to do what it takes!" (O'Hara 1995, 191).

Kristal, Jeremy, Addison, Luke, and the other second wave workers you have met in this chapter have molded a distinctive discipline from the legacy of American Transcendentalism and immigrant-based medical pluralism. As fully fledged adults, Veeda, Rupal, Janelle, and David are starting careers and families; they bear a weighty moral burden to work on themselves and to be productive. In part, this health culture can be used to buffer the demands of work and expand the potential of other spheres of life. However, it can also be used to augment them so that they can perform better than well—at work, in play, and for their families. This group of productive adults may not have invented this health culture—much of that distinction goes to the older cohort in the first wave—but they have embodied it more thoroughly. The next generation, the cohort I will call the "third wave," was born into deep medical diversity; they grew up with the expectation of augmented productivity. Their story constitutes the next chapter.

youth = past turtles reneuting cultural boundaries
- genetic fate / evidence   breaking
    - Education, family, online/offline culture shaping
    (next gen of worries
    (written affirmations in
                            schools etc
questions why there is an understanding of health as
a personal task to manage ie not pments or gove

4   Gearing Up

Babies born screaming
  In this town
Are miserable examples
  Of what happens
Everywhere
  Being Crazy is
  The least of my worries
—Kerouac 1995, "46th Chorus," 47

Cindy Chen and Friends, Crafting Embodied Selves

On the surface, growing up in Silicon Valley is much like growing up
in other urban American places. It is, however, a place distinguished by
daily encounters with technology, a willingness to experiment, and cultural
complexity. Young people draw on multiple cultural traditions and digitally accessible symbols to augment and enhance themselves. Their experi-
mentations can be technical—extending themselves with devices. They can
also transform themselves physically and cognitively through exercise, diet,
drugs, and **body modifications**. The techniques they use can stem from
global immigrant traditions, their own and those of others as well, and
from the marketplace of global popular culture. Access to digital media has
made permeable the boundaries around childhood. Children toy with more
adult metaphors and tasks by connecting with the Internet. Young people
are also subject to the structural changes that have occurred in the adult
work world. The metaphor of productivity and the experience of stress,
products of political and economic individuation, are being learned and

felt by the members of the third wave of change. These digital natives have been born into the world of the new economy, and know no other reality.

The story of the third wave of change, for the youngest cohort, is less about health care than it is about the crafting of the embodied self. The members of this cohort are young, and chronic health problems are less pressing to them than learning how to be in their own bodies. Identities are not free-floating intangible things, but shifting cognitive constructs manifest in physical form. Their bodies are projects in themselves. Cindy Chen illustrates this cultural experimentation with identity and body to define an ever-morphing, deeply diverse self.

Cindy, among the oldest in her cohort, was born in 1985 at the beginning of the digital age. She was born just when consumer computers and "third generation" video games were coming to market, and she was in kindergarten when Tim Berners-Lee wrote the program called "World Wide Web." When Cindy began high school, PDAs and cell phones began to infiltrate her daily experience. Napster made musical file-sharing a reality, augmenting the hot informal barter market in burned CDs. When she graduated from high school, camera cell phones were entering the marketplace. During her time in college, blogs (created in 1998) and wikis such as Wikipedia (founded in 2001) came into widespread use, and Cindy's cohort populated social networking sites (created in 2002). In her youth new services appeared—online phone systems such as Skype (established 2003), Internet-based podcasts (available 2004), and video-posting services such as YouTube (accessible 2005) (see Rainie 2006, 1). The chances are good that as you read this book she will remember only those high school friends that have kept in touch with her through MySpace, Facebook, and subsequent social-networking products.

While still in high school, Cindy Chen sits in her bedroom doing her honors English and advanced chemistry homework on the computer. Photos of her friends, almost all young Asian women, are interspersed with animal photographs and stuffed animals around her bedroom. She also displays athletic awards for tennis and badminton. Her best friends are Tran and Anh, ethnic Vietnamese, who also play badminton, a sport dominated in Silicon Valley by Asian Americans. They have been her friends since elementary school. Along with her mother, and her forays into the Japanese language, they help her establish her identity as an Asian American.

While she does her homework, Cindy is also instant messaging (IMing) her friend Julio, cultivating her social as well as her intellectual life. Cindy never chats online with total strangers, nor do others in her peer group. Friends of friends are possibilities, but such communication is undertaken cautiously. She carefully cultivates her network: "recruiting, colonizing, grafting . . . boundary crossing, activating, pruning" and monitoring her assemblages of friends and near-friends (Gorbis et al. 2001, 55).

She is simultaneously listening to Weezer, an Alternative rock band, whose poster adorns her wall and her computer's wallpaper. Music is not mere background for Cindy and many others in her cohort of emerging adults. Throughout the stories in this chapter music is central to establishing and signaling social identity, and youth experiment with it continuously. Music is the basis for serious identity work for young people, and this is the time of life when most musical tastes are established (Levitin 2006, 232; see also Haenfler 2010). Musical technologies are the most likely medium to be coupled with other devices as young people digitally outfit their environment (Foehr 2006, 8, 18). Computer-based musical systems interface with Apple iPods and other cell phone/mp3 players to create a ubiquitous environment of embodied musical immersion.

Cindy Chen is part of an immigrant family, and that reality shapes much of her identity. Cindy's mother, Joan Chen, is a widow, an immigrant from Taiwan, who works hard in sales at a fiber optics company. She sent her daughters to Mandarin Chinese Saturday school so Cindy and her sister can at least converse with her and the extended family. The girls also learned music and karate, since, as Joan says, "I want them to be strong so they can protect themselves. It's very important, for girls especially."

Cindy is studying Japanese in high school, as did her grandmother in Taiwan, when it was under Japanese control. Cindy is part of an active network of Asian language students at her high school. Her teacher, Robert Jones, is a network architect. Mr. Jones has created a lively Japanese language program. Students have home stay exchanges between San Jose and Okayama. They compete in Japan Bowls, games created by the Japan-America Society that test language proficiency and cultural knowledge, held regionally and nationally. Japanese students also compose a Japanese cheering group for their high school football team (although they are largely shouting out numbers and the names of months!). Mr. Jones comments that he wants "to help students move beyond the sense of 'I am a part of this place,' to 'I am part of a larger world.'"

Making oneself interesting is an essential strategy for being distinctive in the social and career marketplace, and risky behaviors are more entertaining than safe ones. One of the things that third wave youth must do is cultivating themselves for a global, fluid economy in which social capital is generated by being *interesting* and *culturally competent*. These strategies imply some serious management of self and body. It would not be an inappropriate metaphor to say that these young people are building a brand for themselves, which they imagine someday marketing in the new economy. They will be seeking opportunities for networking and entrepreneurship in which they must distinguish themselves. This brand is only partially comprehensible to their elders; they are signaling primarily to each other—for potential mates, cocreators, and coworkers. The brand is coded with information about cultural sophistication, superficial and intimate, marked by clothing, body movements, and modifications.

Cindy's networks in her culturally diverse high school take her to unexpected places. Julio connects Cindy to a cultural segment of San Jose that lies outside of her carefully constructed realm of sports for college applications, academic achievement, and global citizenship. Julio is her online buddy, although they first met in algebra class. He still thinks of her as a potential "cool" girlfriend, since they "connect" through alternative music. He just graduated from high school and plans to become a gourmet chef, attending the prestigious Culinary Institute of America. His father and grandmother live in Mexico, and he is estranged from, but still lives with, his mother in San Jose. Julio has chosen an unrelated African-American-Filipino family to be his "second family." His godfather, part of yet another family, helps him maintain an e-circle of friends who make up his garage band. Yet another set of his friends are the FNH (Freak Nasty Ho) warriors; with them he plays miniature golf, bowling, hockey, and video games, especially Marvel vs. Capcom, a series of fighting games. He enjoys defining his group of friends as "fun loving criminals" who illicitly **street race** Honda Civics.

Gaming and Internet chatting, technologically mediated experiences, stimulate him as little else. As PEW Internet researcher Amanda Lenhart has noted, "Creation is not just about sharing creative output; it is also about participating in conversations fueled by that content" (Lenhart et al. 2007). Seeking sensation, as an end in itself, is part of this generation's media experience (Foehr 2006, 11). Through technology, Julio creates a social existence that is embodied differently than that of the older cohort. He is more comfortable connecting socially through devices than his elders imagine possible. He finds intimacy in instant messaging that he says is lacking in face-to-face and telephone encounters. In such chats, one can really be oneself. Silberman writes of another teen, a sixteen-year-old from Santa Clara, who echoes this sentiment. This young man struggled with his queer sexuality, not knowing quite how to conduct himself with the men who attract him. Referring to such an object of affection he says, "If he was online, I could tell him how I *feel*" (1998, 120). Online formats are more genuine to Julio, less influenced by the nuances of spoken communication. Interestingly, Julio has chosen a profession, cooking California cuisine, favoring fresh ingredients and influenced by global food traditions. This craft is deeply rooted in the physical body, in spite of Julio's preference for a cyber existence.

One of Julio's friends is Nat, who is "not actually but might as well be Mexican." Nat "eats" Mexican and imbeds himself in Mexican friendship networks. Julio finds nothing unusual about adopting a cultural identity unlinked to ancestry, an unforeseen consequence of living in deep diversity. Dee, slightly older than Julio, an immigrant from Hong Kong, articulates a common philosophy: "I guess I would say that most people, like myself who grew up here have a struggle with identity. . . . I work with teenagers from different backgrounds . . . immigrant people, who went through what I went through. I like to be creative . . . using my imagination, art, challenging norms, society, rules, regulations, morals. . . . I like exploring, experiencing. I am always meeting new people, finding new places to go, trying something new, different, every day. . . . I feel like I never fit into certain categories." Fitting into categories neatly is more difficult in a culturally complex milieu. Cindy, Julio, and Nat find themselves extending beyond their "ancestral" categories to which they are born; they extend, prune, and modify those identities with new practices.

The Children of Silicon Valley

Members of the first and second wave mixed and matched cultural modules, creating new hybrid practices. The third cohort is beginning to open the modules, the "black boxes" of culture, and create new practices that go beyond expected ancestral identities and predictable youth cultures. The third wave is experimenting with boundaries with an abandon that perplexes and even frightens the older cohorts. The boundaries at risk are many. They play with ethnic identity, decoupling the link between ancestral and enacted identity. They test the exchanges between personal and professional activities, play and work. They constantly test their own agency, mixing risky behaviors with healthful ones, trying to find the balance between enhancement and excitement, augmentation and danger. Some of these identity and risk trials are part of the culturally appropriate age behaviors of children, and especially teenagers. However, other behaviors are rehearsals for adult activity. Some of these young people are already in the workforce, if only as interns or apprentices. These future Silicon Valley workers, if they remain in the region, will be more information literate, and more digitally savvy than their elders, even those just a few years older.

Young people in Silicon Valley have a distinctive setting in which to play. For the last half-century, Silicon Valley has been a global magnet for high-technology expertise. For families that have resided in the Valley for many generations, multiple connections bind them to the technology sector. Parents are engineers, elder cousins are marketers, and siblings act as creative interns in tech companies. For families newly moved to the area, high technology itself—or work in service to that sector—is why they came!

The stories of the children of the Valley, whether they are six years old or twenty-three, invoke several serious questions. As the people in this coho themselves note, *they are the future*, and they bring a different sensibility to that future. They are native to the experiments first established by their elders—the first and second waves of change in the region. Experimenting with self, enacting deep diversity, toying with life stages, and seeking intensified productivity are taken for granted as embodied disciplines for this cohort.

Luis and Davis, Experimenting with Risk

Inviting, mitigating, and managing risk are important activities among youth. Many of the risks of modern society are invisible—few inhabitants of South San Jose know they are sending their children to an elementary school built on a Superfund site. Indeed, the nature of risk is open to interpretation depending on one's place in the larger social structure—unequal distribution of knowledge can change one's awareness and reaction to hazard (Beck 1992, 21–22). Luis chases risk, since he is preparing to embrace an entrepreneurial existence. Living at home, working for his mother, his economic risk-taking is buffered, so he experiments with other activities—extreme sports and technical tinkering. Davis, a bit older, has experienced more of the consequences of physical risk taking, and experiments with alternative practices. Instead of actively participating in risky adventures, Davis is quietly creating business opportunities associated with outdoor living and skating. These two young people are experimenting with that tenuous balance between avoiding risk and seeking excitement.

Luis was born in Argentina and moved to the United States at nine months, nineteen years earlier. He texts his girlfriend to make sure she sells her stock as it is going up, and troubleshoots his friends' computers. When he wanted to build websites, he learned the necessary program, called around until he found someone to host the site, and "just experimented." He wants to be an entrepreneur, to own a business like his parents, so that he will have autonomy. "People earning their paychecks may be making as much," but they cannot control as much of their lives and be *flexible*! Not for Luis is "Oh, I only have five days of sick leave, only have five days of vacation leave left." The corporate environment shaped by the older generation, or even the university classes designed to funnel workers into the companies, does not appeal to him. He is confident that his ability to communicate comfortably and work with technology will open up the doors he needs. Luis rejects institutional structure and moves in and out of college, which he sees as redundant and largely useless. Luis says, with pride, that his friend going to Stanford comes *to him* for technical help. He dropped out one term after getting a "weird sickness" and missing classes in order to race his car. Luis makes himself interesting pursuing intense experiences such as street racing, skiing, snowboarding, rappelling, and "finding new stuff to do." Like others in his cohort, Luis prefers "sharing, staying connected, instantaneity, multitasking, assembling random information into patterns, and using technology in new ways" (Rainie 2006, 1).

Davis, like Luis, was once an avid camper, hiker, and climber. Then he had a survival experience that went sour. "That was a difficult time, because I was really disillusioned with wilderness. I didn't realize how untamed . . . and that I wasn't invincible." Davis started having panic attack episodes and found it difficult to leave the house. He tried to work on himself, adopting a **vegan** diet, but he wasn't sure how to do it and ate almost exclusively carbohydrates—pasta, tortillas, cereal, rice. Underweight and malnourished, he recovered with the help of nutritional and psychological therapists. Now he publishes a skater-oriented music journal. He works with a recreational equipment co-op and goes to Hewlett Packard to give talks about outdoor recreation, staying fit, and "staying straight on the work, and also having time to free yourself of that and stay creative." He has worked his way through the tangle of risk and self-experimentation to find a path that works for him.

Mastering skateboards is linked to a particular lifestyle that accents risk and self-discipline. Skating "makes you have to deal with yourself. It makes you go, 'Okay, it looks easy. Now try it.'" Skating not only involves mastery of emotions and body but also communicates "cool" to an admiring audience. Skating was one of a cluster of exciting activities Davis Fisher cultivated. He published an underground newspaper, although, to his surprise, his teachers and the principal actually applauded his involvement!

Luis toys with open-ended entrepreneurial activities; his risks are well within the local cultural celebration of individual agency and invention. Luis's embodied perils include adventuring in the wild, transcendental natural play that fits his experimental frame of mind. When those outdoor adventures became too risky, Davis converted his desire for thrill to skateboarding, and then buffered the risk even further by publishing for the skateboarding subculture. He managed the emotional consequences of his risk-taking with the help of an ecosystem of caregivers. Davis retuned his body through fitness and diet. He converted his risky passions to professional experiences, creating content for online publishing.

As social theorists Ulrich Beck and Nikolas Rose suggest, risk is a situated calculation. Risk is inherent in the "entrepreneurial spirit" that intensified in the last decades of the twentieth century, the time period in which Luis and Davis grew up (see Beck 1992; Rose 2007). Demonstrating the ability to take risks builds a particular sort of cultural capital. However, it is also calculated based on knowledge that is unevenly distributed. The embodied consequences of risk have not yet been experienced by young people who imagine themselves "invulnerable." Davis learned the lesson that he is not immortal the hard way, so he must find new arenas in which to test himself and build his brand as a risk-taker.

John Carter, Living on the Straight Edge

Eighteen-year-old John Carter is also a gamer and digital native. At the edge of independence from his father, and his father's insurance, John must weigh his risks carefully. "Health is how many points you have," says John, slipping into a gaming metaphor. The fewer ailments, "coughing . . . all the way up to cancer . . . AIDS, the very dangerous stuff," the more health points you have. In this video game of life, John has had experience with a serious point deficit. At eleven, before he moved to California, he began to have epileptic seizures. At the hospital, "My Dad was crying. It was the first time I ever really saw my Dad crying. I was like, 'Oh, this is serious.'" For a while he was a celebrity at school; he was "that kid that died." A roller coaster ride of changing medications "messed with his metabolism" and caused him to go from "hummingbird to buffalo." John gained a significant amount of weight and became "a fat kid." His parents did not want him to play video-games or other experiences that might be potential epileptic triggers.

Obesity is a risk factor structurally connected to wealth and class, for money can buy the most nutritious calories. The poor buy the food most likely to lead to obesity because it is inexpensive. Obesity is also a matter of subjective interpretation—even supposedly objective measures, such as the body mass index, obscure the fact that the ratio of fat to muscle can differ based on age, fitness, or gender. Body image exists amid a wealth of cultural messages that range from a pathological loathing of visible body fat, such as the sentiments experienced by John, to impassioned celebrations, such as Sir Mix-a-Lot's "Baby got Back" ("I like big butts").

Slowly John was weaned off his medication as the seizures stopped, but he was left with a consciousness of his metabolism that continued into his adolescence. Moving to and from California, bouncing between his divorced parents, he used his cross-country moves to reinvent himself. When he had new friends, he decided he might as well "be different . . . a new me." Even though his father and diabetic aunt smoke and eat unhealthful "Irish" food and super-size portions, John experiments with healthy living. John tries to "eat less" and "eat smarter." He cooks "rice and fish" at home instead of going out to eat "a big old bucket of ice cream and an extra large fries." Like more than 30 percent of his age mates, John uses the Internet to get health information (Lenhart, Madden, and Hitlin 2005, 9). Using Google's search engine to find "healthy recipes" off the Internet, John changes his lifestyle. He starts to work out, and the weight begins to melt off. The changes were so dramatic that one of his teachers worried he that had bulimia! He continues to monitor his eating, stopping when he starts "to feel full." John does his sit-ups at home, sometimes wishing he could afford the gym. Video games are no longer off limits and provide the central metaphor of his bodily management. He is racking up those health points.

At the first opportunity, he moved into a mobile home with his younger relative, consciously creating a more healthful environment. John searches for a better apprenticeship as an electronics technician intern that would include insurance. Without that safety net, he plays his daily game of living cautiously. He takes no risks while riding his bike (no racing or trick riding), avoids sick and potentially contagious people, and uses instant messaging to maintain his social life while avoiding physical contact. His "backup plans" include asking relatives to help him should he really need it, which is "a really reassuring feeling."

John is **Straight Edge**, a movement that advocates avoidance of sex, drugs, and alcohol. This movement has many facets, ranging from militant veganism to a more moderate philosophy—that the body should be left to experience the intensity of musical and political passion without chemical interference; it's straight, with an edge. Symbolized by an "X" (once marking underage patrons in punk rock venues), members of this movement call themselves, sXers, or Straight Edgers (Haenfler 2010, 31). This movement requires that adherents embody particular disciplines, eating primarily healthful, largely vegetarian foods, avoiding alcohol and mind-altering drugs, and practicing sexual abstinence. The movement has "a variety of meanings for individual sXers, including purification, control, and breaking abusive family patterns" (Haenfler, 2006, 37). It has been an active movement for nearly thirty years and endures in spite of peaks and valleys in its popularity.

Several of the people interviewed in London affiliated themselves with Straight Edge and explained its philosophy in ways that illuminate John's choices.[1] Greg says, "I am still proud to be Straight Edge; . . . it's a really productive thing that I did." Greg says that it allows him to put his own stamp on his experiences, rather than being affected by "drugs, or an urge that I can't control." Caffeine, however, is a common exception. "You can have caffeine and be Straight Edge—loads of people do." Straight Edge provides a flexible, and coherent, way to manage his body.

John's experiences with chronic illness have sensitized him to his body. The Internet and his network of friends provided new fodder for interpreting his bodily states and managing them, overcoming some of the "unhealthy" socialization he had as a child. His age-specific poverty and lack of insurance provide inflexible constraints. John cannot afford to take the physical risks that Luis does, or use complex and expensive devices that Luke uses to manage himself. So he turns to social institutions, such as the Straight Edge movement, that foster simple living without being socially and culturally dull.

John can be edgy and risky in his music, his philosophy, and his sense of self, without the added expense of alcohol and drugs, both legal and illegal. However, such drug abuse does exist among John's age mates. Mel, for example, became a meth addict. His father was a "workaholic. He was just work-work-work-work-work . . . a real grouch." Mel joined Narcotics Anonymous and started a twelve step program to work on his addiction, with a strict sponsor. His sponsor tries to get him to reframe his negative self-perceptions. Like the Straight Edge movement, Narcotics Anonymous creates a competing world view to allow people to be edgy but not over the edge.

Alan Davidson, Modifying Bodies, Experimenting with Pain

People in the third wave begin to shape the strategies they will adopt in their adult years. They customize their practices, selecting a distinctive set of practices including body modification, foods, nutraceuticals such as vitamins and extracts, and using prescription and nonprescription drugs. John uses music rather than drugs to be edgy. Davis experiments with vegan and vegetarian living. Debbie Carson's son, Derek Rogers, experiments with homeopathic and Chinese remedies. Staying focused and in tune with the body is a challenge; people's attention is drawn in multiple competing directions. When multitasking is the expected norm, staying in touch with the body is a demanding discipline. In such a case, pain itself can be used to focus concentration and manipulate cognition.

I was attuned to this self-management style by a young programmer who uses the pain of multiple body piercings to take his awareness out of his head—where his world is coding software—and back into his body. With this in mind, I visited Alan Davidson, a tattoo artist, chef, business owner, and keen social commentator. Like the other forms of embodied cognitive manipulation we have seen—taking drugs, practicing Straight Edge, eating, or exercising—physically modifying the body spans generations, bridging together the worlds of youth and adults.

Body modifications are multifaceted phenomena, fascinating to anthropologists. Obviously embodied, they signal belonging to certain social segments—Straight Edgers and modern primitives. Straight Edge identification is signaled by marking oneself with an "X"—shaving it on the scalp or tattooing it. Tattoos signal a degree of commitment and authenticity instantly communicable to peers (Haenfler 2010, 38). Modern primitives, epitomized by San Francisco's Fakir Musafar, search for spiritual growth by piercing, tattooing, scarification, and body deformation (DeMello 2007, 47, 191–95). Practices can range from tattooed tribal patterns that encircle the wrist to experimental sadomasochistic sexual practices. Associated with nomadic high-tech professionals who wanted spiritual grounding in new practices, the movement was particularly potent at the turn of the millennium (see Mizrach 1997, 141). Modern primitives literally mark their bodies to indicate their affiliation with the movement. Such tribal tattoos do not make much of Alan's practice in recent years. In fact, removing these patterns generates business for him now. He notes, "I'm covering up those things like crazy now."

Tattoos can be "flash"—generic designs—or customized to reflect a person's particular path (see Photograph 8). Increasingly, tattooing is moving from a standard set of designs to more customized, private statements drawing on a "cultural pastiche" (DeMello 2007, 115, 266). Clients find images to reflect their own musical tastes, spiritual paths, or identity constructions. Customers tell Alan, "I want this and this and this to represent my journey." Identities change, and these transformations are rewritten on the body. The tattoo "party animal" may be fine for an eighteen-year-old but inappropriate for a young career woman or mother at twenty-five. Alan will not tattoo spouses or lovers' names. In light of modern American kinship, the dyadic bond of marriage is too fragile for something as permanent as a tattoo. It is lines of descent that matter; parents and children remain intact bonds. People memorialize their deceased ancestors, family, and pets. Tattoos can be "covered" or altered, integrating an old design into a completely different one, when the direction of one's life changes (see Photograph 9). Tattooing's reputation is still "rough," but it also has its own cable television network program. There are tattoo parlors for vegans, for families, and specialty artists who do only the proper Polynesian "shorts," waist to thigh designs, done with ritual and dignity. The modification itself is a cultural message.

In addition to the content of the tattoo, clients experience an intense alternate bodily reality in the process of getting the modification. Pain is a critical part of tattooing. When people come to Alan for a tattoo he tells them to expect pain and "prepare for the worst." If you don't "they start seeing little spots and they are hitting the floor." Some of his clients sleep through the tattooing process; others find it the most intense experience imaginable. Once one tattoo is done, however, people think, "That is not as bad as I thought!" He doesn't believe you should try to avert the pain, "because you're joining a club and you have to abide by all the rules." Some people get tattoos in less sensitive spots, the exposed skin of the arm. Other "people I know get tattoos in the worst places, because that is how they deal with life. . . . Getting tattoos is easier than dealing with emotional pain." One girl got a massive tattoo with roses and fire saying "Revenge," expressing her angst at having every one of her relationships fall apart. She told him, "I'm centering all my energy into this tattoo," instead of lashing out at other people. When you are getting tattooed, you are surrendering yourself to the artist. One woman, who is in a major video game company, says she doesn't get vacations, so body modification is her "way of relaxing," of going to a place quite distinct from her everyday work world.

Augmenting Self

Modification, itself a technical metaphor, alters the bodily experience of self. Yet there is another technoscientific metaphor, *augmentation*, that even more profoundly shapes the bodily conceptions and practices of this third wave cohort. Fitness can be seen as an augmentation, improving particular parts of the body for particular purposes. Luis builds an arsenal of risky practices to augment his entrepreneurial state of mind. Derek Rogers augments his body in the gym in order to look a certain way on stage. Cindy Chen consciously fortifies her college applications with participation in badminton, seen as the sport of Asian students, augmenting her identity work and keeping active while pursuing a career. Digital natives have grown up with augmentation as a master organizing principle for those who created the technology around them.

In the earliest days of Silicon Valley, it was assumed that the goal of the infant information technology sector would be to produce artificial intelligence, replacing humans with machines. Doug Engelbart, among others, realized that empowering humans with technology, *augmenting* them, was not only a more reachable goal but also one consistent with the countercultural sentiments and experiments of the time (Markoff 2006, 43–48). Much of the technology of Silicon Valley is built on the principle of designing devices that will augment human experience, performance, and productivity. Augmentation can be chemical, technological, or cultural—you drink Redbull,[2] imbed your network in Facebook, or learn to be competent in Japanese popular culture.

The advantages of augmentation must be balanced against the potential risks, and that is a juggling act young people must master. In particular, the search for more energy, more focus, and more productivity leads to experimentation. Caffeine is the obvious substance to augment such states—in forms ranging from the ubiquitous liters of diet Coca Cola to Jolt Espresso, or new flavored Jolt drinks that add ginseng, taurine, and vitamin B complex. Caffeine and other stimulants are the drugs of choice for knowledge workers, even though that may actually impede cognitive function for complex and novel tasks (Reid 2005, 17). Although this is contested by those who look at its biochemistry, those doing sustained concentrated work are measurably enhanced by it. Caffeine is widely available in Pepsi-sponsored vending machines in regional high schools or offered gratis in high-tech work spaces.

This should not come as a surprise. Chocolate, coffee, tea, and, later, colas have been intimately connected with the birth of modern work practices. Wage labor and industrial work practices broke tasks into distributed components, deskilling guild crafts and creating repetitive monotonous labor. People had to regulate themselves to the clock. Caffeine is particularly effective at sustaining performance on such tasks. Its use also went hand in hand with the temperance movement, replacing the ubiquitous ales and beers with stimulants (ibid., 15; James 1997, 42; Weinberg 2001, 126).

There are, however, other forms of neural enhancement in the classrooms and cubicles of Silicon Valley. One hidden source of embodied productivity is the nonmedical use of prescription stimulants. Many of these drugs are prescribed for the treatment of ADHD, attention deficit hyperactivity disorder. These pills flow through networks, from people with prescriptions, real and falsified, from biomedical channels to those who use them. The younger the onset of use, the more likely the practice is to be addictive (McCabe et al. 2007). In the national surveys that have been done, approximately 40 percent of the users say that they use it to increase productivity; 23 percent use it to stay awake, with undergraduate men being the heaviest users (Novak et al. 2007; McCabe, Teter, and Boyd 2006; Sussman et al. 2006).

"Increasing productivity" is too broad a phrase to describe what these drugs do. They help users focus on problem solving, and increase the flow of adrenaline. A Silicon Valley teen comments, "It's like tunnel vision: You just zone in" (Patel 2005, 1A). In California the abuse of prescription drugs is increasing. Fifteen percent of eleventh-grade high school student used such pharmaceuticals without prescriptions (Mercury News Wire Services 2006). Seven percent of Palo Alto high school students said they had tried Adderall, Ritalin, or Dexedrine at least once. Quoted in the San Jose Mercury News, Becky Beacom, of the Palo Alto Medical Foundation, notes, "It's like mental steroids. Students think they need that extra edge to get them into college" (ibid.). Students themselves classify these drugs in the same category as Redbull or caffeine. Managing schoolwork, after-school activities, and social networking at the level these students feel is necessary requires augmentation.

This particular style of augmentation continues into the adult world of knowledge work. Whether using Adderall, Ritalin, or Provigil (Modafinil, used to treat narcolepsy and ADHD), a recent survey of *Nature* subscribers revealed that roughly 20 percent of the readers use these drugs to augment their memories, enhance focus, or improve concentration (Reuters Health 2008; Maher 2008). Overwhelmingly, even nonusers believed that the use of these prescriptions improve their performance. Four-fifths of the *Nature* subscribers believed that adults should be free to take the drugs if they choose. A third of the subscribers also said that, while in principle they objected to the use of these drugs in minors, they would give them to their own children if other children had access to them (Maher 2008, 675).

The use of "cognitive enhancers" foreshadows future cosmetic neurology, analogous to cosmetic surgery (Chatterjee 2007). Such illicit use by adults sits side by side with a new generation entering the workforce who have been diagnosed with ADHD and continue to need prescription drugs to function at a high level (Read 2005).

Bryant Evans, Cognitively Diverse

Where augmentation and cognitive self-consciousness are integrated into everyday life, a new form of identification is emerging—**cognitive diversity**. In Silicon Valley, this can be seen in the way in which the epidemiological identification of Asperger's syndrome with that particular place creates a kind of regional pride. In 2001, *Wired* magazine ran a piece which suggested that Silicon Valley was an epidemiological hotspot for Asperger's syndrome, a form of autism that has been dubbed "the geek syndrome" (Silberman 2001). The story was picked up in national magazines such as *Time* and in the local media (Seipel 2002; Hull 2004). This narrative suggested that "math and science" genes were being concentrated in the millennial generation, presumably biologically linked to the technological elite of Silicon Valley. These highly intelligent young people would be "geeks," lacking social skills and the ability to read other people but imaginative and innovative.

While there is no evidence of such genes epidemiologically, the idea was embraced and even celebrated. In addition, jokes began to be made about the ADHD generation being uniquely positioned to multitask, at least on Ritalin, in spite of medical evidence to the contrary (Siklos and Kerns 2004). What is important in this discussion is that a new form of diversity, cognitive diversity, joins the many other matrices of difference at play in the Valley. The Valley's cognitive "others" began to be referred to as "Indigo children," a reference to a New Age story in which synesthetes, people with unusual sensory perceptions, represent a new stage in human evolution. Casual references to gaming and anime motifs reinforce this identification as young people casually ask each other about their particular "superpower."

Bryant Evans epitomizes such a person. His family pioneered the computer industry. He has been diagnosed with OCD (obsessive-compulsive disorder) and social anxiety disorder. Bryant has two great passions, robotics and Egyptology. These interests are supported by local institutions. NASA and Lockheed work with schools to support interest in robotics, while the Rosicrucian Order's Egyptian Museum houses a large collection of Egyptian antiquities and employs interns. He participates with his alternative high school's science fiction club and has organized a philosophy debate club. Bryant self-identifies as someone with "serious" mental differences. He describes the social interaction of his high school using World War II as a metaphor, noting, "High school is a World War II situation. I am Switzerland. I'm a neutral country, not opposed to anybody and I have good ties with just about everybody out there. I speak everybody's language. I know how to talk to people. I know how to talk to the homeys. . . . I know how to talk to the hackers, 'What's up, dude?' I know how to talk to the intellectuals, because that's my first language, really. And there are just so many people." Bryant's assessment harkens to the many youth "subcultures" that define embodied existence—"goths, theater kids, athletes, skaters, computer and band 'geeks,' hip hoppers, emo and metal kids, among others" (Haenfler 2010, 4). Their distinctions overlap with ethnic and class markers but also reflect cognitive and behavioral orientations. Each identity group reifies and advertises itself through food, clothing, music, and chemical augmentation. When the members of the third wave cohort speculate on how their minds and bodies work they create cognitively based identities such as "geekiness."

Jocelin and Mark, Imagining Gene-based Selves

Genetics is another criterion for building identities as people imagine their future selves, adding to social complexity. In Silicon Valley, arguably a concentration of people with scientific training, genetics is also transformed into a moral mechanism, explaining particular health "weaknesses." Genes are not viewed as binding constraints. Among the teens, explanations of genetic inheritance resemble religious accountability—a tendency noted by scholars of American epistemology (Finkler 2005). The genetic sins, or salvation, of the fathers provide a framework in which people can engage in free will to tinker with fate. Jocelin, a young Filipina, sees the genetic dice of her family loaded against her, saying, "My grandpa passed away when I was eighteen, and he died from . . . chronic heart [disease]. . . . So that had an effect on me, because I felt like that's pretty common in my family." So she changed her practices, explaining, "I definitely want to be more healthy future-wise." She builds a set of practices, eating breakfast, taking multivita-mins, drinking more water, and, with utmost difficulty, eliminating sodas. She is healthy now, but, projecting herself, with her genetic burden, into later life she modifies her daily life. Jocelin points out, "It's more of a future thing."

Mark Winters too carries genetic risk. His mother has diabetes, and he is overweight. He is a college graduate and lives with his parents, holding down two jobs, waiting to get a professional job as a residential counselor. He knows that exercise is the key to his weight management, and that his family is "an addictive personality family." He has a Straight Edge friend who has helped him see sugar as his own personal drug, but he craves it anyway. He *knows* he should exercise more but is just "very comfortable with inactivity." Diets will not work for him, and as a waiter he scorns people who come into his restaurant wanting special changes to the menu. The diet fanatics annoy him. Mark says, "God, the Atkins people drive me crazy!" He is irritated by their pickiness and wonders why they bother going out to eat, even though he knows that is often the only way to efficiently juggle work and social life. Nonetheless, he rails at fad diets and struggles to find his own path to weight management—his own "sin of the fathers." His mother watches him, worries, and tests his blood sugar with her glu-cometer. The pieces of his network of health accounting—genetics, eating, exercising—remain out of sync.

The ways in which Jocelin and Mark account for the causes of ill health and underlying foundations for health are part of a larger agenda of iden-tity work. Genetics is one factor, but karma, agency, and even cultural purity all play a part in defining who they are. It is not novel to suggest that health states are integral to identity. Cancer survivors, people with HIV, even the obese form distinct identity groups, especially where sup-port systems encourage such identification. These Northern Californians have adopted health identities that support self-tinkering so that they can remake themselves into healthier, more productive people. The cognitive and genetic identities that Bryant, Jocelin, and Mark have made contribute to the overall pool of deep diversity in the region.

Otaku, Anime Fans, at Home in Deep Diversity

In 2002 I applied philosopher Charles Taylor's idea of deep diversity to Silicon Valley (English-Lueck, 117, 37). So many people of different cultures reside together that the sheer quantity of intercultural interactions produces a new form of social intercourse. The differences are not just surface ones but reflect deep variation in how the everyday world is viewed and enacted (Redhead 2002a; Taylor 1993). The children of Silicon Valley are growing up in such a world, interacting in neighborhoods, schools, and malls to produce a pastiche of cultural behaviors.

Cindy, Julio, and Nat are part of that immersive cross-cultural environment, as is Janet, a self-confessed anime addict and GSA (Gay-Straight Alliance) member. She says, "Culturally, I am a blend of American and Chinese, although mostly I make my own culture." This hybridity does not mean that the embodied powers of racism and discrimination have disappeared, but "it is not as obvious as it was in, like, the 1950s; it's more sophisticated now." She navigates her network creating two kinds of family—her "blood family" and her "spiritual family" with whom she feels a connection and a tangible trust. Deep diversity can lead to interesting cultural experiments as youth draw on multiple social worlds. Lacey, Janet's classmate, combines immigrant Ethiopian and Goth identity, a fascination with vampires and dedicated community service. Lacey, however, plans to socialize her future children into traditional Ethiopian practices.

This cohort is making a conscious effort to shape a moral compass to help navigate the diverse range of choices. Media, such as televised and Internet-based Japanese anime and written **manga** (graphic novels), provide content for navigating complex moral choices. Silicon Valley high school students draw on Japanese pop-culture, spirituality, and stories of heroic sacrifice to broaden their repertoire of values. The genre of anime resonates with a longing for augmented hidden power that is part of the gaming cosmology of digital youth. Anime creates a global fantasy landscape, similar to the **social imaginary** discussed by anthropologist Arjun Appadurai, "full of worlds that are essentially mental (and often technological) constructions" (Napier 2005, xii, 293). In these mythical productions, protagonists and antagonists struggle with issues that speak to Silicon Valley youth. Many anime plots are set in schools. Hybrid identities abound. Characters strive to understand their own alienation; their bodies often transform from one organic form to a different, often a technological one (ibid., 23–26, 37).

Silicon Valley children and teens construct their cognitive categories from watching their elders and friends work and heal each other, and they learn from Asian morality tales in anime and *manga*. Anime struggles with the same tensions as Californian transcendentalism. On the one hand, technology is pervasive, and the boundaries between the human and the products of human engineering are ephemeral. Machines enhance and augment, often intimately, the human characters. The *manga* character Edward Elric is the Full Metal Alchemist who is partially transmuted into a cyborg, augmented by auto-mail, a full metal prosthesis. His brother Alphonse is completely transmuted. Their quest is to master alchemy, to fix the "mistakes" Edward made as an immature alchemist, and restore Alphonse to his natural body (Arakawa 2002).

Although the technology in them is exciting, many *manga* and anime echo Shinto imagery, in which nature is sacred. There is a deep longing for *nature* in anime plots, especially vanishing nature (Napier 2005). For example, the anime character Chihiro is the central protagonist of *Spirited Away* [*Sen to Chihiro no Kanikakushi*], directed by Hayao Miyazaki. This film is an Academy Award winner, at the forefront of global anime popularity. A self-absorbed young girl, Chihiro, leaves modern-day Japan and enters a ghost-world in which she must earn her freedom and rescue her parents, who have been transformed into pigs. She works in an unearthly bath house managed by the witch Yubaba. She helps a river *kami* to remember his true draconic self, which had been lost to pollution and urbanization. Only through hard work, self-discipline, and spiritual love can Chihiro transform herself, her family, and friends (Clements and McCarthy 2006, 606).

A typical Miyazaki story, *Spirited Away* is about the holistic metamorphosis of "what was lost" to "what could be," but only if the protagonist is brave, respectful, inquisitive, and clever enough (Napier 2005, 124, 53). The transformation motif of anime characters is not just physical or merely spiritual, but a fully integrated event. These lessons are not lost on their Silicon Valley *otaku* disciples.

Otaku create fan fiction, combining existing anime universes with their own stories to explore sexuality, friendship, family, loyalty, and good and evil (see Haenfler 2010, 114–15, 120). Through art posted to DeviantART, and stories posted to Internet blogging sites FanFiction.net or Live Journal, *otaku* shape alternative bodies. Takero, who is seventeen, built his personal network around anime and Japanese language, finding that by doing so he is part of a group of "friends a lot smarter than me" who help him with his schoolwork. Tan, another *otaku*, is Vietnamese, ethnically Chinese, but considers himself "Japanese a little bit," since most of his identity work is rooted in anime. He is president of his high school's anime club, writes fan fiction, and studies formal Japanese. Anime interest groups may be supported by their schools, as was Tan's, which has a faculty-sponsored club and a library that purchases *manga*.

The Internet offers fans a chance to create a complex world of fan fiction, accessing and subtitling Japanese-only animation and creating mashups of *manga* and anime images dubbed with music drawn from a variety of genres. By creating a participatory media culture, young people consume and produce content in formal and informal economic exchanges (see Ito 2008, 9). Anime *otaku*, "Japanime geeks," see the art form as intrinsically productive, augmenting skills in drawing, digital prowess, and even cultural competence, drawing on the assumptions of Japanese culture.

Diane and her family left China for Canada when she was six. Her father is an engineer and that drew him to Silicon Valley, leaving her with a sense that she is a "little bit Chinese and American and Canadian." She identifies with the themes of Japanese anime, saying, "A lot of people who see that would say it's kiddie stuff, but if you really watch it, each film has a deep meaning inside. It's about friendship and human striving in life." Childlike media formats and adult themes are intertwined, so it is increasingly difficult to discern the worlds of children from the worlds of the adults.

Restaging Childhood

While children and young teens can easily be classified as minors, the upper end of the spectrum is less well defined. Young people are gearing up for adult responsibilities for production and caretaking. They can enter that stage at seventeen or at twenty-five. Again, I find myself thinking of traditional Chinese Confucian life-staging, in which a young male is not really a man until he has solidified his education and career and begun a family. In Silicon Valley, in a similar fashion, attending undergraduate and graduate universities delays the onset of those fully adult obligations. Start-ups blur the lines between educational experiences and creative productive work as university friends become coworkers. The high cost of housing in Silicon Valley delays the creation of a separate household not dependent on parents. Luis is an entrepreneur, a sometime student, but he also lives in his parents' home. John Carter is the adult caretaker of a relative only a bit younger than he, but he is still an intern. A critical turning point occurs at twenty-two or twenty-three when parents' job-based health insurance policies no longer cover the nearly adult children. Competing cultural definitions of life stage convey mixed messages to children who are not sure when they have grown up.

The key to the transition to adulthood is productivity. The years of childhood and adolescence are used to experiment with processes designed to augment creativity and foster efficiency, with parents to buffer them financially, at least in the middle class. This exploration is done in a deeply diverse environment in which mythologies, bodily practices, and self-identification draw from many different cultural wellsprings. The children of Silicon Valley see their parents, elder siblings, and mentors augment themselves, articulate an ethic of hard work, and make every effort to be productive.

In American society, children are caught in an interesting paradox—they are separate from adults in many ways, yet utterly intertwined and dependent on them. Childhood is constructed as a "mythical landscape," a special time and place in the cultural imagination. Segregated by age, children are turned into "islands" in which children's spaces are isolated from adult geography. Like small landmasses in the oceans, children are surrounded by adult activities and spaces, yet they have a distinctly different experience of their own. The "free spaces" of children, however, are intensely monitored by adults (Gillis 2008). Children and adults do interact, however, in intimate household settings and formal institutions such as schools, churches, and recreational arenas. Some of these institutions are public; others reflect the privatization and the proliferation of new market niches in everyday American life. In Silicon Valley, companies have a strong presence in public and private education, supporting particular programs and activities (English-Lueck 2002, 95). If children are islands, then they are supplied by the adult mainland, and the habits and proclivities of adult taste flavor their provisions.

However, the distinction of childhood is made more problematic by immersion in digital technology, central to the world of this third wave. Young people in this cohort, from the smallest babies to those in their early twenties who have not yet fled from the nest, are digital natives. The younger the children, the more complex and technologically saturated their reality. Their parents grew up in a more stable and lucrative work world, but these children will most likely have to reinvent themselves many times over the course of their lives as workers. Rolling down the aisle at a chain grocery store, these children see alternative medicines side by side with over-the-counter pharmaceutical products. Unlike parents and grandparents who could comment on a television program only to those in the room with them, this cohort can video capture the content, manufacture captions, make voiceovers, actively create and post media collages on the Internet to be viewed by their friends. Their ecosystem of devices, provisioned by the adults, is informally traded among the children. Their lives are thick with electronic instrumentation. Computers are a given. More than 90 percent of teens are computer users, and 85 percent have used either mobile devices or computers to communicate: emails, instant messaging, or through social networking sites such as MySpace (Lenhart, Madden, and Hitlin 2005; Lenhart et al. 2008). Some 64 percent have created their own content (Lenhart et al. 2007). Even among the lowest income households, nearly half of the families in California use computers (Fox 2003, 1–4).

These young people are sophisticated about how social networks can be built, manipulated, and modified. They are not necessarily more adept at relationships than their elders, but they are more conscious of the instrumentality of relationships and more comfortable with the easy affect that comes with weak ties. Even though they may have deep and rather narrow passions, those interests draw upon a global smorgasbord of cultural practices. They have eaten each other's cuisines, borrowed each other's words, and adopted each other's identities, building a cultural competence, from the ground up, that their elders can barely comprehend. The process of becoming digitally competent comes early.

Pet Projects

Sociologist Anthony Giddens, who has long examined the interplay between social structures, institutions, and individual agency, reflects on the cultural production of contemporary self-identity. He casts the creation of self as a "reflexive project" in which people project themselves—bodies, appearances, demeanors, sensualities—into the future and subject themselves to particular regimes to achieve that goal (1991, 75–99). It is an act both conscious and shaped by a plurality of social institutions. Teenagers in Silicon Valley are working on their own *projects of self*, turning identity work into a constant stream of projects, many of them technologically mediated.

These young people send instant messages, order products, and Google to search for health or homework information at the same time they are playing music, watching television, and text-messaging friends on their mobile phones (Foehr 2006, 1–10). The term "multitasking" draws too much attention to the tasks themselves, rather than the milieu in which the activities are situated. These devices are connected to particular social worlds, specific *contexts* in which the person is imbedded. An instant-message text may trigger recall of a particular situation. When Manny receives a message about music from Rachel, who is in Manny's third period government class, that context reminds him that there is an assignment due. While parents and teachers use email, and still think it an innovation, teens think it is for "old people" (Fox 2005). Rachel's grandmother sent her a present for her birthday; she should email her a quick "Thanks." She has seen a particular television program many times, and only a few of her favorite parts are still interesting; the rest of the time it fades to the background but may provide a bit of content to stimulate texted conversation with her friend. It is not really the information that matters, but the connection, cementing the social ties of friendship (see Horst and Miller 2006, 89). Music evokes an emotional context; Rachel is plugged into a song that expresses the grief she feels for the father who passed away. Multitasking is less the act of switching between device-based tasks but more the importance of navigating the interconnected fields of meaning.

These children begin their lives as digital natives on websites like that for **Neopets**, training virtual pets, armoring them, and competing in the Battle Dome. Some 23 million people, primarily children (slightly more girls than boys), play in this animated universe (Belden 2006). They feed and care for their pets, which will sicken and die if neglected. Players explore Neopia, and create fan fiction, and write to each other through a filtered channel of communication called Neomail that limits conversation by age. Children collect rare treasures, hoarding and spending Neopoints in a brightly colored reflection of consumer capitalism. Players can lose points gambling, gain points through wage labor, and invest points in the stock market. Barter and even theft are possible. A not so subtle instrument for inducting children "into consumer culture," Neopets is also "a venue for kids' mobilization and productive activity . . . learning complex skills of social and economic negotiation, exchange, leadership and achievement outside the narrowly predetermined structures of achievement set up by formal educational contexts" (Ito and Horst 2006, 6–7). Gathered around the computer—discussing gaming strategy, the theft of Neopoints because of the sharing of a password, quibbling over control of the mouse, and petting their purchased plushy Neopets—friends engage in important social play.

As my youngest daughter proudly tells me, this site prepares her for the "real world;" *she* understands mortgages better than her parents. As she drifts from Neopets to Gaia, an anime-themed social gaming site, playing also prepares her for interlacing face-to-face, alternative, and digital worlds seamlessly. Like her peers, she is transliterate—adept in multiple media—layering avatar upon subplot, creating multiple new habitats out of digital media, print media, television, and creative play. This pastiche constitutes the social worlds inhabited by the digital natives of her generation. If her social spaces are islands, then they are ones with very busy interconnecting digital ferries.

Sunny and Hettie Schwartz, Embodying Structures of Individual Performance

Children are situated in social institutions—families, schools, and retail establishments—that teach values, narratives, and practices that discipline creativity, productivity, and bodily management. These institutions, like the workplaces of their parents, have been subject to the structural changes of the last few decades. Individuation, in the form of personal empowerment, is manifest at schools and in families as well. Children must be prepared for their future lives, and educational and commercial venues must help parents stay focused and productive. Preschools and retail sites abound to manage children for working parents, and they support their socialization. Commercial and nonprofit organizations promote lively "participatory arts." Children can glaze ceramic pieces at the small chain shop Petroglyph, take craft classes at Michael's Arts and Crafts, or perform in nonprofit immigrant cultural organizations such as the Firebird Youth Chinese Orchestra, where young people learn to play traditional instruments such as the *erhu*, *pipa*, and *ruan*. At a local community center, John XXIII, young people from a local high school's Vietnamese club perform for the elders. At an Indo-American center in Milpitas, diverse Indian languages are spoken and both Bollywood and traditional Bharatnatyam dance classes are offered (Moriarty 2004). This participation in "the secret artistic life of Silicon Valley" involves not only children but their parents as well. Hewlett Packard, Varian, Quantum, 3Com, and Cadence, among many others, informally nurture creativity among the "hidden" musical, visual, and performing artists that work in these companies (Alvarez 2005).

Dancing, singing, and exercising are tools in the kit used by young people as they experiment with their bodies' appearance and energy levels. They can also reflect serious identity work if those activities give them a connection to their cultural tradition or one with which they want to cultivate a link. Shalini Shankar, in her nuanced ethnography of the "Desi," Indo-American teens, describes the complexities of creating a performance of Indian dance at a Silicon Valley high school to represent their "diversity." Beyond the obvious difficulties of selecting a dance from India's many ethnic groups, there is the micropolitics of who chooses the dance and the style. One girl comments that she wants to "join a dance" but not with the "snobby" girls who "live way up in the hills" overlooking the Valley. Beyond this problem of class, the dance chosen is not traditional but "filmy," in the Bollywood style, with "slutty" dance moves that may offend families. Dance is a physical activity, but it is also an embodied identity act (Shankar 2003, 214–16).

Some of these acts of socialization are deliberate and set a pattern later seen in teens and adults; other messages are unintended. The Schwartz children, Sonya (also known as Sunny) and her little sister, Hettie, live in an artistically rich environment. Their parents are successful attorneys who have consciously cultivated a household that is educationally cultured, inviting their children to become connoisseurs of the world's diversity of art, food, and music (see Darrah, Freeman, and English-Lueck 2007, 57–60). Their parents model a strong work ethic, even though they have a family rule of not "bringing work home." But conversations about the need to negotiate with colleagues and opponents at work, made during evening homework sessions, socialize the next generation. Daily intellectual disciplines are intimately integrated into everyday life.

The Schwartz daughters go to performing arts camps in the summer, a convenience for working parents and a source of important life lessons. Sonya's group performs a medley, singing and dancing for a convalescent home for the elderly. Her mother, Linda, says that this has been a "real eye opening experience for Sonya, really good for her." She had not been exposed, face-to-face, with much suffering, and that was a "growing experience for her." Civic engagement is as much a part of this household as the cultivation of humor, music, sports, books, and food. Families provide guidelines: school-based affirmations shape other social contracts.

Affirmations—short statements designed to shape ethics and attitudes—

are used at home, in school, and during work to reinforce conscious self-management. These artifacts guide youth so that they can craft a particularly American self. Signs in Sonya's middle school are aimed at disciplining a moral self with "life skills" such as "flexibility, courage, humor, friendship, caring, integrity, organization, curiosity, common sense, perseverance, respect, responsibility, patience, effort, problem-solving, cooperation, and initiative." An inspirational picture notes that we "all smile in the same language." Other posters ask, "How are you smart?" Are you gifted with cognition oriented toward "logic, music, world, self, picture, people, body or nature?" This sentiment fosters a particular kind of self-reflection and lays the groundwork for thinking about cognitive diversity, in which differences in thinking and feeling can be viewed as potential assets. Across the Valley, in a less affluent section of the county, a school poster, produced by the Santa Clara County Network for a Hate-Free Community, depicts a group of teenagers all of different ethnicities, captioned, "We don't stand for hate. We stand together" (see Photograph 10). Whole networks of teens resonate with this message, and work on themselves to make it true.

Sonya and Hettie Schwartz study Hebrew and attend the Sunday school associated with their reform temple, where they learn the history and culture of American Judaism. Their public and religious education promotes conscious reflection on self, morality, and daily practices. Of course, aphorisms have a long history of shaping action, as Sonya's Sunday school activity illustrates. After studying the venerable Ten Commandments the students generate their own list:

Thou shalt always wear sunscreen.
Thou shalt use a Kleenex when blowing the nose.
Thou shalt not leave the toilet seat up.
Thou shalt not smoke.
Thou shalt not feed the goldfish too much, just a pinch.
Thou shalt learn to type.
If you take a tree down, plant another one.
Thou shalt play basketball and swim.
Thou shalt not put muddy shoes on the carpet.

In her middle school classroom Sonya is asked to make three affirming statements about herself, and she says, "I am fluent in another language (Hebrew). My family usually eats dinner together. I think of myself as a smart person." As she enters her math class, two questions are written on the whiteboard. "What is your game plan to accomplish your goals? How are you going to keep track of improvement?" These problem-solving approaches, one of the life skills listed above, will play a critical role in shaping how these children manage tasks, including health-related tasks.

These educational aphorisms mirror the normative statements of workplaces, values brought home to families. At the Internet company Yahoo, workers are told that they should value "Excellence" and be "committed to winning with integrity." They are to be "flexible and learn from our mistakes." At the same time, they are to laud the value of *fun*. As the company says, "We believe humor is essential to success. We applaud irreverence and don't take ourselves too seriously. We celebrate achievement. We yodel" (Yahoo! Inc. 2008). Yahoo also has "thou shalt not" aphorisms. The company adds that they do *not* value arrogance, sloth, vaporware, discrimination, a stick in the eye, 90 percent (performance), or decaf—the sins of the twenty-first century. Google proclaims ten things they know to be true, including "Never settle for the best" and "You can be serious without a suit," proclaiming a fun-loving culture of work that "fosters a productivity and camaraderie fueled by the realization that millions of people rely on Google results" (Google Inc. 2008).

Sensitized to this use of proverbial sayings, shorthand for communicating moral knowledge, by my own ethnographic work among intellectuals in the People's Republic of China, I am struck by the ubiquity of the affirming slogan. These sayings discipline workers, family members, and future citizens, creating a schema, a formula for encouraging a creative, tolerant, and self-monitoring future workforce. This same strategy is used to discipline health practices. Called "affirmations" in the health education sector, they include a variety of sayings designed to promote sustainable dietary and exercise regimes. Used to motivate dietary change at Kaiser Permanente, or praise women exercising at Curves, affirmations, using the dearly valued power of positive thinking, begin to take root in the children of Silicon Valley. Affirmations are an integral part of working on self.

Jessica Maglaya, Subject to Individuation

Members of the third wave are subject to the burden of individual empowerment, and draw on many diverse cultural resources to try to navigate the structural changes they have inherited. The structures of work, family obligation, and self-care are less clear. Managing this ambiguity creates stress, which they experience intimately as the source of their malaise. Jessica Maglaya came to the United States from the Philippines as a toddler. Jessica is twenty-four, an immigrant daughter who lives with her parents, but she is just past the age when she can be covered by their health insurance. Like John Carter, she avoids sick people and has become a "bit of a germaphobe." She also tries not to do "stupid stuff" that might endanger her.

Jessica's mother is diabetic and she associates food directly with health, saying, "What you put in your body determines how well you are!" But food also flavors identity. Especially at family gatherings and cultural events, she worries about eating Filipino food, declaring, "I can't really get away from all of the fatty foods because it's part of my culture. . . . I look at my culture and there are a lot of unhealthy foods." Nonetheless, she is careful when she can be, living mostly on rice and vegetables.

Her aunt in the Philippines sends her articles on health, sometimes accompanied by a birthday card—how to "lower cholesterol and blood pressure, de-stressing, dealing with PMS, old people health-related problems." She monitors her parents' health, gives her mother her medications, and angrily tells her father not to smoke. In fact, she won't hug him again until he quits smoking; the boycott has lasted nearly six years now. Each time he starts to approach her, "Dude, you're a smoker. No!" She practices beliefs that differ from her family's. While being deeply medically diverse adds to her repertoire of health tools, it also complicates her ability to create sustainable practices.

Jessica has larger health goals imagined for her future. Even though there will be difficulties—Jessica is a lesbian—she really wants children. She sees herself in training for this time, saying, "And, I want kids. . . . I want to have my body ready for kids. Because I want them!" So she creates a regime of practices, including stress management, healthful eating, lining up professional work that will provide financial stability and decent insurance. Jessica draws her notions of health, food, family, and work from multiple cultural sources including her immigrant relatives and her diverse peers.

Jessica Maglaya identifies stress as a major source of malaise in her life, and pinpoints its origins in her social relations at work. Being queer and Filipina, stress emerges from intercultural conflicts, and from having "straight men hitting on her." It also comes from work pressures, struggling through, in her case, the quagmire of studying social theory in school. Jessica, with a disgusted tone, comments on her books, "They increase my stress because I start to panic. I read through them and I say, 'Oh my God, Oh my God. I don't know some of this stuff!' And I panic. And my stress level rises. And then when that happens, I am like, 'Oh my God! I need a Tylenol!'" She works in an attorney's office and comments, "I know that when I am under all that stress and pressure I tend to get sick more. And I'm trying to stay away from sick people at work. Because I know a few of the attorneys are getting sick. I try not to touch any of the things they touch or not stay in their vicinity too long because they know I am prone to getting sick and I am really stressed out." She believes stress is the trigger for her acne and her migraines; this explanation accounts for her frequent use of Tylenol and prescription pain medication.

Stress can be viewed in one of two ways. Stress can be a quantifiable and measurable biologic state, one induced by irreconcilable social pressures. It can also reflect folk models of explanation, providing a broad meaning-laden category that accounts for why people get sick or well, linking causes with outcomes. In a study done on the San Jose State University campus, anthropologist Darrah and his team found that students and staff alike used a holistic and all encompassing set of explanations for being healthy, including nutrition, exercise, and sleep. Chief among the culprits blamed for illness are work and time-compressed "stress" (Darrah, Monzel, and Turner 2007). In my own ethnographic experience, stress is constantly being cited as the cause of illness, just as Jessica Maglaya identifies it as the source of her anxieties, acne, and migraines.

Stress is an explanatory blunt instrument, as malleable in its meaning and application as a belief in **animism** or **animatism**. Animism is an explanatory belief system in which natural and artificial worlds are imbued with conscious spirit entities that must be addressed to avoid misfortune and illness. In an animistic explanatory system, gods, demons, and spirits are the basis of physical misfortune. Celia referenced such spirit beings in one form of medical *qigong*, as an explanation for illness. Most people, especially young people, talk about stress as if it were animatistic. Animatism is the belief that inanimate forces, which lack consciousness, can manifest themselves in everyday life and cause misfortune. Luck, *qi*, *élan vital*, and energy are all examples of such animatistic concepts. In everyday usage, people speak of "stress" as such a pervasive inanimate force. Stress is a metaphor to reflect profoundly subjective states of imbalance, not only to refer to the measurable biomedical effects of adrenal cortisol hormones.

In the subjective conception of stress, the ordinal quality of having more or less stress is the basis for experiencing worse or better immune response. Stress is the reification of social demands, work intensification, life pace, and the pressures of self-management. A consequence of the logic of self-empowerment, stress is inseparable from the larger system of production that values such self-generated action. In his discussions of **somaticization**, medical anthropologist Kleinman notes that somaticized emotions are "moral stances in an ideologically constructed behavioral field." He notes this in the context of studying depression in premarket Socialist China, in which depression would be read as political critique. In a similar way, people who were caught up in the "great age of business" in the late-nineteenth-century United States experienced neurasthenic symptoms of fatigue, dizziness, and weakness. Such a diagnosis gave them permission to rest (Kleinman and Kleinman 2007, 472). Using "stress" to account for disease allows people in Silicon Valley a modicum of social critique and a means to mitigate the morality of work pressures.

The third wave draws on a rich ecosystem of practices, beliefs, and tropes, fueled by immigration and transcendental experimentation, to find a balance point between being risky and safe, cosmopolitan and dull. These choices are inscribed on their bodies. They try to find the boundaries for childhood and adulthood, in spite of the many competing formulas given to them by parents, peers, and institutions. They augment themselves with fitness practices and neurochemical prostheses, and use metaphors from the worlds of anime and superheroes to describe themselves. They struggle with explaining the misfortunes of body with diverse etiologies, ranging from food to stress, cognitive differences to genetic karma, and to find practices to counter these causes. The question remains, however, why they should feel it is their individual burden to account for illness, manage their energy levels, and remain productive. Even though they are, or have recently been, dependent on their parents and other institutional support, they have learned that those supports are not always reliable, and that ultimately health—and every other aspect of embodied existence, is their personal responsibility. The individuation of responsibility is part of a larger social pattern in which the structures of health care have been reconfigured. These structures of institutional care, including health care delivery, work, and retirement, have undergone deregulation and decentralization, and have become a complex maze that people must navigate. These changes have taken place throughout the United States, but they are easier to spot in an expensive place like Silicon Valley, where class translates so obviously into health.

[handwritten marginal notes:]
ill or aged ... of workplace → people as obsolete if not productive
also racial exclusion in economic down-turns
shift in care responsibilities away from state
communities of fate — pooling of similar health groups
restructuring of retirement healthcare commodity or figure?
eh as no support + wanting to be useful still
— how to age well
— inequalities of living well
region, local etc
structural ← work etc
violence ←

5 Structural Failure

Tree over and down
Its root-rot clear to the air, dirt tilted
Trunk limbs and twiglets crashed
On my mother's driveway—her car's barricaded
Up by the house—she called last night
"I can't get out"

—Snyder 2004, "Winter Almond," 53

Matt Turnstall, Intensive Self-Care

Matt Turnstall, born in 1950, suffers from a plethora of chronic conditions. In his youth he was in the Navy, performing search and rescue missions. He was shot and bears the scars. He had asthma, but the prednisone he was prescribed made him "blow up like a balloon." When his vision became blurry, he was diagnosed with diabetes. He went to classes and learned to test his blood glucose and to administer his insulin. Matt's feet began to feel numb. This neuropathy prevented him from feeling his toes, so when he broke them at work—Matt is an electrician—he didn't stop working. His toes became septic and were amputated. His prosthetic foot caused him problems. The year 2001 was the dot-com crash in Silicon Valley, and the ripples from that implosion were felt throughout the local economy. Matt remembers, "I lost my job and 9/11 happened and the job was history."

Then his kidneys started to fail. Faced with grim medical choices, Matt opted for home **dialysis**. His dextrose solutions are color-coded. Green-labeled solutions are 2.5 dextrose, and he uses ten liters a night to flush his system. If he gets overweight, he switches to red, 4.5 dextrose, which "will drain a lot of water out of me." Matt explains, "It's a daily routine with me. I have to get up every morning, get on the machines, and then I have to restock the machines. As soon as I get up and dismantle it, I put everything back the way it should be, so tonight all I have to do is plug in this, a peritoneal catheter. It was installed by surgery." It is a tube coming out of his side that drains his peritoneal fluids. "I just plug myself into that, and I'm on my way. It's like ten hours a night, but it drains me and fills me, and then gives me a break for an hour and 50 minutes. I can get out and do whatever I want." He has to keep his solutions stocked, crowding his small home. He must test his peritoneal fluid for infection to be sure he is not getting peritonitis, and he keeps all the antibiotics he needs in case that happens.

With kidney problems, he has to be careful to avoid foods with potassium—such as milk or bananas. Impaired renal function also leads to greater levels of parathyroid hormone, and weakened bones; so far he has broken two ribs. Matt has been on the list for a kidney transplant for five years and could have a wait of six months to two years more. He would not ask any relative for a kidney, "unless I was dying or something." Meanwhile, his self-care is intensive.

The noise of the machinery bothers Matt's wife, so he tries to schedule his dialysis around her work schedule, and he worries about her. The specifics of caregiving have changed. Caregiving no longer involves seating the elders "by the fire, bringing them an occasional cup of tea, and waiting for them to die." Instead it means administering medication, operating complicated devices, preparing special foods, and coping with medicalized depression. Care also requires navigating labyrinthine bureaucracies and handling complex financial arrangements (Roszak 2001, 121). Adding alternative healing practices to biomedical care requires even more expertise.

Although Matt is adept at taking care of himself, being a caregiver for others falls disproportionately on women; daughters and wives provide 57.6 percent of the care for elders, while sons and husbands provide 32.3 percent. Only 13 percent of elder care comes from social service agencies (Coward, Horne, and Dwyer 1992, 24). Caring for others may also be a significant obstacle to taking care of one's owns chronic disease burden, as well as a source of anger and depression. Extended care can lead to "role strain," a weariness that comes with being the caretaker wife, daughter, or husband. Caretakers feel isolated, which makes recovering from depression and bereavement that much more difficult (Aneshensel, Botticello, and Yamamoto-Mitani 2004, 423).

Matt sometimes works small jobs as a subcontractor. The time he spends in dialysis and fighting his own fatigue prevents him from working more than four hours at a time. This employment supplements his meager retirement income. Without the jobs, his income would be 30 to 40 percent lower. While Matt and his wife might be able to sustain their household more easily in a less expensive place to live, they must hustle to stay in the Valley. In spite of the ecology of ills that plague him, Matt's self-assessment is positive, "My health is pretty good right now. I'm a little bit tired." Matt knows he is getting care, and he can still care for himself. He is fortunate.

Placed in Jeopardy

An unintended consequence of the close linkage of employment and health care is that those who are underemployed or unemployed—by becoming chronically ill, aging out of the workforce, or both—become marginalized. Matt's layoff and struggle to keep his home illustrate how economic instability adds to the burden of chronic health care. The health problems of the people relegated to the economic fringe are intimately connected to economic structural flaws. After decades of converting "regular" employees to contingent labor to improve the bottom line, health care benefits are scarcer. People who are not in the paid and insured productive workforce suffer poorer health care access, experience barriers to health self-management, and undergo more stress.

The stressors of work, work-family articulation, and busyness exacerbate problems in health management. Although estimates vary, 54 percent of the Valley's adults are overweight or obese, although that number drops if you factor in the more affluent areas of San Mateo County (Fenstersheib 2007, 16). Some 20 percent of adults in Santa Clara County are clinically depressed (Health Research for Action 2007, 44). While the chronic health burden of Silicon Valley is not particularly high—the educated workforce is actually unusually healthy by national standards—access to health care is complicated by the instability of the economy.

That volatility is felt among the professional class and the other 60 percent of workers alike. The dot-com bust that began in 2001 lasted a full five years, resulting in hundreds of thousands of Silicon Valley workers being unemployed or employed with substantially reduced wages and benefits. Recovery from that event was undermined by global recession in the final years of the decade. At the height of the boom, in December 2000, local unemployment was 1.3 percent; by November 2009 it had climbed to 11.9 percent (Public Policy Institute of California 2004; 2009a, A1). In the first crash, median household income fell nine thousand dollars. Latino- and Asian-headed households were hit most dramatically by the recession, and seven of the top twenty occupations in the region paid less than a living wage by 2007 (Auerhahn et al. 2007, 9). Local hopes for a green-tech economic upswing, although not gone, seem to belong to a more and more distant future (Carey 2009b, C1). In the United States, the probability that a person's family income could drop by 50 percent or more has gone from 7 percent in 1970 to 17 percent in 2002 (Hacker 2008, 31). These economic factors, both microscopic and macroscopic, are critical health stressors, whose effects interact with and are played out in the workplace, the home, and the community at large (Pearlin et al. 2005, 210–14).

The pattern of boom and bust leaves an economic legacy that plays out in the daily lives of its inhabitants. Silicon Valley is an expensive place to live.[1] This volatility produces intense uncertainty for the workers, especially among the tenuously employed contract and temporary staff. Of all states, California has the highest churn rate, a measure of job mobility and turnover (Benner 2002, 47). Within California, Silicon Valley experiences intense churning at each boom and bust cycle. Jobs, especially mid-level ones, require more frequent employer switches, geographic mobility, retraining, and shortening job tenure, and more frequent wage fluctuations. More and more people are self-employed, the most vulnerable of tenures (Henton et al. 2008, 7–9, 50). With classic Silicon Valley optimism, this is seen as uncertain territory, but one that could hold unforeseen opportunities. After all, this scenario increases the number of economic and technological experiments going on and, therefore, the possibility of the next radically new but efficient generation of profit-making products. The social situation demands social and cultural flexibility, while people experiment with the fabric of everyday life to survive, but at the expense of constant stress and uncertainty.

Having health benefits is critical to the employers themselves for a number of reasons. It is an essential recruiting tool, especially for high-value knowledge workers. Employers need the "benefit" of health to recruit and retain employee talent. This competition is even more intense among silicon places given the proliferation of employers outside of the United States; it is part of the "quality of life" that attracts globally mobile workers (see Asheim and Gertler 2005, 298). Improved health means improved productivity. The evidence is mounting that *managing* the chronic disease burden, rather than denying it, translates directly into less absenteeism, presenteeism, and higher worker "quality" (Goldfarb et al. 2004).

Silicon Valley's experiences mirror a larger set of changes in the work world. Even what constitutes employment has shifted, as more and more workers are contingent "contract," temporary, or self-employed workers (Sullivan 1999, 457). Downsizing was an overt corporate strategy in the 1990s, boosting stocks by "streamlining" the workforce, producing a new category of highly skilled, flexible contract workers (Barley and Kunda 2004, 10–12). This is particularly true in Silicon Valley, where employment is tiered: company employees with full benefits, high-functioning contractors, and poorly paid temporary workers likely to be denied such benefits (English-Lueck 2002, 30; Barley and Kunda 2004, 312). There is a reason that Rupal, with his new-born daughter, feels so grateful for his benefits. Finding job-based health coverage in Silicon Valley is increasingly difficult.

The burden of empowerment is felt keenly when it comes to managing health. Vast numbers of Americans are not insured. Ten percent of Silicon Valley falls into that category (Henton et al. 2009, 34). This metric masks the greater numbers of underinsured who have pre-existing conditions, or must provide copayments beyond the reach of many workers, especially contingent workers (Barlett and Steele 2007, 593–95). Employers, insurers, and health care organizations have shifted the onus of health care to individuals; care is a problem to be managed within their families. This shift is framed in discourses of individual responsibility, promising individual people that their costs would go down if they engaged in "good behavior."

Of course, health care has undergone structural changes more massive than would be indicated by mere changes in rates of insurance coverage. Health care is "at the epicenter of economic insecurity" in the United States (Hacker 2008, 187). Biomedical health care is the portal through which we see the American values of risk management, faith in experts and technology, and reliance on the invisible institutions of government. The ways in which risk is understood and translated into insurance premiums has been shifting through the beginning of the twenty-first century.

In the Great Depression, consensus could not be reached on how to create a one-payer, governmentally based health care system. Physicians, insurers, and employers were hostile to government health insurance. As a pragmatic alternative, the government advocated privatized insurance. Blue Cross was the pioneer in this form of "private social activism," creating a scheme by which risk was pooled across a broad segment of workers. Through a series of practices such as forming insurance pools, marketing, designing rating and underwriting systems, and evaluating and compensating losses, insurers evolved to have two competing functions. One task was to manage financial risk for investors, while the other was to provide health coverage for their customers. These two functions have become increasingly incompatible (Heimer 2003, 299–301).

Having a large pool of relatively healthy workers is essential to a functional model of health insurance; the broader the pool, the smaller the probability of risk to the insurer. The dynamics are similar to having an aquarium. A large aquarium has sufficient water to stabilize the variation in pH and temperature, while a smaller, less expensive aquarium is subject to rapid fluctuations in water quality, damaging the fish. However, a large aquarium also requires a complex set of filters, rockwork, and structural supports that a small aquarium does not need. Choosing a large aquarium is a better long-term choice for the health of the aquatic community, but it is less likely to yield short-term benefits. Similarly, a broad pool of healthy workers stabilizes the risk, but the competitive nature of private health insurance pools led to fragmenting the worker population into many smaller and less stable "pools." These small pools were less stable, but also "cheaper" to start, maximizing profit.

In 1948 the Supreme Court ruled that health insurance benefits could be included in collective bargaining (Numbers 1997, 275). The workplace became the site for obtaining and maintaining care. Medicaid (Medi-Cal in California) and Medicare evolved out of this fundamental structure in 1965. However, in the 1970s several structural changes occurred in the insurance industry that changed access and costs. Rivals to Blue Cross had already "poached" insurance customers, offering lower-risk groups discounted premiums, and eventually Blue Cross itself changed its **risk pooling** practices. Then, the 1974 Employee Retirement Income Security Act contained a clause that allowed companies to pay for their workers' health costs directly, through "self-insurance," bypassing the state regulations directed toward other forms of insurance. Self-insurance proliferated, but with unintended consequences. Self-insurance and micropooling made better sense for investors but undermined the delivery of health care.

Small companies did not have enough workers to pool the risks effectively, so that healthier people could offset the cost of aging and chronically ill workers. Blue Cross changed from broad pooling to hypersegmentation, and the risk of becoming ill was being borne increasingly by families themselves as costs increased and services dwindled. Insurers create "communities of fate," in which the healthy are pooled together and pay lower premiums with smaller deductibles and the less healthy pay more (Heimer 2003, 298). In smaller pools, the inclusion of riskier workers drives up costs to workplaces, which pass those costs onto employees. In California, average health care costs to individual workers for job-based health coverage doubled from 2000 to 2006 (Auerhahn et al. 2007, 11). The reformulation of risk into micropools has shifted the burden of health care onto individuals (Hacker 2008, 7). However, small risk pools led to a "death spiral" of rising costs, partially the result of separating the inexpensive healthy from the expensive chronically ill—driving up overall costs (ibid., 151). Late-twentieth-century employer-based health insurance structures are not sustainable, either for the organizations or the individuals paying premiums.

The ongoing debate about reforming health-care funding in the United States continues into the second decade of the twenty-first century. Private insurance companies, often partnered with workplaces, are the premiere option, at least in the imaginations of consumers. Public options, such as the existing Medicare and Medicaid programs, tap into discourses of government growth, control, and taxpayer burden. At the heart of the debate are the complex and multilayered narratives about health. Is health care a commodity? Is well-being a right? Is the right freely to design and sell health products more central to American values than the individual's right to health care access? Once Roosevelt had turned away from the public option in the Great Depression, the obstacles for creating such an option have grown steadily more formidable. The structural linkages between workplace, insurance, and health access are too deeply imbedded in practice and policy. While changes may occur over the next decade, they are unlikely to be revolutionary. Workplaces remain a primary portal into private health care, although an increasingly privileged one. Meanwhile, ongoing changes in worker status and workplace obligation make individual workers more vulnerable.

In the United States, 6.8 million workers over fifty are self-employed. Some of them have accumulated considerable assets, particularly if they have been running their own businesses for many years. Newly self-employed workers are much less likely to have such assets—36 percent compared with 55 percent. They are also unlikely to have pensions (Zissimopoulos and Karoly 2007, 61, 73). If they are not among those with saved assets, such self-employed workers are navigating a grim fiscal reality. These "lone wolves" must keep working—working contract to contract. In Silicon Valley, whether they are old or young, this group is growing faster than the rate of new full-time jobs at firms (Henton et al. 2008, 5).

The children and grandchildren of Silicon Valley workers face other structural shortfalls in accessing care. In Silicon Valley, nearly 98 percent of young children are covered by public or private health insurance (see Auerhahn et al. 2007, 11). These youth, however, are moving into a work world that might not give them the benefits their predecessors expected, and their health access will be correspondingly less secure. They are already endangered by their own health practices—overeating, sedentary living, interpersonal violence, and self-destruction.[2] Mental health facilities are in short supply for children and teens, as well as seniors, in spite of a robust ratio of physicians in Santa Clara County, 345 per 100,000. The normal recommendation is 145 to 185/100,000, but the services of that surfeit are directed to those with insurance, not to those most in need (Health Research for Action 2007, 35–44).

Global flows that both generate and displace work in Silicon Valley have unintended health consequences. Traveling and migrating from around the world, workers bring their diseases with them. While the United States has a tuberculosis rate of 4.6 out of 100,000, Silicon Valley's rate is 13 out of 100,000; more than 90 percent of these people with tuberculosis are foreign born (Fenstersheib 2007, 31–35). Living at a global crossroads complicates the pattern of disease in Silicon Valley.

Elderly immigrants have the lowest rates of health literacy. Monolingual Spanish, Chinese, and Vietnamese speakers over sixty-five have especially high rates of health illiteracy (Health Research for Action 2007, 82). There is a serious shortage of health practitioners in gerontology, even fewer who are bilingual or have the skills to work across cultural barriers. Few practitioners understand the value immigrant seniors place on herbal medicine or the participation of family (see Health Research for Action 2007, 35–37). Seniors can wait more than thirty days for a response from practitioners (ibid., 83). Some 78 percent of seniors rely on family and friends to be caregivers, and 25 percent of them are themselves caregivers—that most stressful of social roles (ibid., 89). In Silicon Valley, people over sixty-five struggle to stay afloat economically.[3] Life is not particularly easy for the older residents of Silicon Valley, financially, emotionally, or physically.

Being elderly is a deeply medicalized life stage. You do not just age, you enter a "state of deficiency" and increased risk (James and Hockey 2007, 147). From the point of view of public health, the oldest citizens of the Valley are the most medically vulnerable. Eighteen percent of older Santa Clara County residents have been diagnosed with diabetes, compared with 14 percent of the adults born after World War II and 13 percent of younger adults (Fenstersheib 2007, 12). Maintaining work and self-care with this disease burden is difficult. Retiring from work adds new dimensions to disease management.

Ben Jensen, Retired in the Cat-Bird Seat

The need to keep working is reinforced in high-cost-of-living areas such as Silicon Valley. The particular configuration of entrepreneurial and small business work in Silicon Valley carries its own constraints. Workers at a national laboratory or a large corporation, such as Hewlett Packard, experience their approaching retirement differently from the people working in the complex ecosystem of small businesses. Ben Jensen was once a manager at a prominent high-tech defense contractor and is now long retired. Ben has fully partaken of the medical riches of the region. He was one of the participants in a Stanford study that identified Type A and Type B personalities in relation to heart disease. He was able to get a pioneering neurologist to handle his first stroke. He keeps his insurance information at hand and keeps meticulous records of his own medical "numbers." His physician tells him to monitor his numbers and it they "get high," to "start watching yourself and your diet." Ben keeps asking his physician if he has to stay on the medication. To the affirmative response Ben replies, "Okay, you're the doctor."

Ben's experience in a stable, large company is different from those who are in the more volatile entrepreneurial sector. As companies appear and disappear, and workers move rapidly from one job to another, the traditional framework for retirement savings is undermined. The 300,000 people in the cohort born after World War II are expected to retire in Silicon Valley by 2018; they face an increasingly insecure future (Henton et al. 2008, 50).

Other Silicon Valley workers find local retirement difficult. They have developed strategies to navigate the pitfalls of retirement, including moving away from the Silicon Valley area for a less expensive, more sustainable later life elsewhere. They can leave. California, traditionally, is a revolving door state; people at retirement age come to retire there, and others leave when work is done (Walters 2002, 46). However, Silicon Valley is particularly cost-intensive, and more Anglo-Americans between forty-five and sixty-five, and Latinos of all ages, are leaving the Bay Area and California for economic reasons (Swift 2008). This is not an easy decision.

It is difficult and expensive to retire in Silicon Valley. To understand the interaction of work, or postwork retirement, and health we must turn to the cohort born before World War II, a generation earlier than the first wave cohort. The elderly in Silicon Valley, as elsewhere, clearly illustrate the difference between those who are wealthy and those who are not. While this rich-poor gap matters at other ages too, the consequences of inequality show up sharply in the ability to age well or ill. After sixty-five a new bureaucratic maze complicates the already stressful world of chronic illness, caretaking, and self-management. For those with resources, and the ability to draw on a lifetime of work tools and disciplines, such navigation may be relatively easy. In contrast, those aging without those skills and assets will find the changes difficult.

Some of the transitions simply come with age—being elderly brings new health concerns, costs, and bureaucratic choices. As they age, Americans must rethink what they are going to do with their extended life span, and they are reinventing the last decades of life. At the same time, the shifting economic reality means that retirement from one form of work may not mean withdrawal from work itself. Like Matt Turnstall, retired workers work less. For some, economic necessity requires them to continue to work simply to survive; for others, those years can be a time of service, rather than mere recreation. They direct that work to the care of others and themselves, but they still work. Caregiving itself has changed and demands constant effort. Access to high-quality care, and the ability to provide it, become one of the great divides between elders who fare well and those who fare poorly.

Dan and Annie Dansen, Silent in Silicon Valley

Dan Dansen identifies with the Silent Generation. He had read Neil Howes's book *Generations*, and he affirms himself to be one of "the good dutiful kids that have gone along trying to keep that all going." At the same time, Dan did live through the transformations of the sixties and seventies and comments, "We were half a generation behind the Flower Children, but we could kind of identify with the Flower Children, in a way. That's what brought in the New Age." He calls himself a "grail seeker," someone who wants to use his retirement to heal the world. His imagery is partly drawn from his years of association with Sequoia Seminars, a community that seeks to resolve science and Christianity through reflection and thought. At the same time, he doesn't see his generation or himself as "postmodern," like the age groups that followed him. Dan asserts, "We're still modern in the sense that there is ... an overarching story, a model that ties it all together. The world may have gotten very complicated, and there may be all these competing submodels" but underneath the complexity Dan is certain that he can figure out what is necessary and "get in step with it."

Dr. Dansen is retired from a long and distinguished career in systems integration, at the forefront of the development of aerospace technologies. He worked at several key laboratories, public and private, and spent much of his time "in advanced development groups. There was a lot of proposal writing. When proposals come, you've got sixty days or ninety days to prepare a proposal and, if you didn't work yourself to exhaustion and lost a proposal, then you would think, 'Well, if I had worked a little harder, maybe we could have won.'" Work was "all encompassing." He left with fourteen boxes of materials, thinking that he would be consulting. His postretirement career did not take the direction he had anticipated, so he threw away 90 percent of the material, keeping only mementoes of key milestones, such as his work on ion engines.

Dan had found a different direction. He explains that his "vocation in religious circles means calling or something that you feel pulled to do." He does not want to simply fill his time, but create meaningful social change. Dan wants to apply "the systems engineering process" to other areas of society, as a "solution discovery process for all sorts of social purposes." The dilemma may be water management or another issue, but Dan wants to continue to contribute. He is not even sure he is in retirement. Dan points out, "What I'm struggling with here is being retired and self-financed. The traditional boundaries between work and not work have kind of fuzzed up. I'm not seeking any monetary rewards from it right now."

His wife, Annie Dansen, is much more pointed. "He's not retired. No, we've got friends who have retired and shoot, they go to China!" Some of their "systems buddies" move in and out of work, but for Dan it is "all consuming." When Annie shattered her knee, she was unable to continue taking care of the details of life that allowed Dan the freedom to devote himself to his work. Instead, he needed to take care of Annie and keep the household going. These tasks used up most of his time, although he was still able to prepare and deliver a major paper on systems applications. Many of his friends were leaving the area; he felt more and more isolated in his pursuit of his intellectual vocation. Many of his friends found the high cost of living outweighed the intellectual richness of the region. Without his friends, burdened by expenses, and sobered by caretaking responsibilities, he found that Silicon Valley's pull grew less strong. With the siren call of a more affordable "nice, woodsy place, with a pleasant little garden," Dan and Annie move to the Carolinas.

Dan Dansen is part of an age cohort whose birth-years range from 1922 until the end of World War II. Those born in the second half of that range, like Dan, had one foot, often as leaders, in the social revolutions of the first wave discussed in the second chapter. The earliest members of this cohort were active in that war, while the younger participated in Korea or Vietnam. Their cohort appears to esteem both compliance and innovation; traditional social roles are to be enacted, but may require moderate editing (Zemke, Raines, and Filipczak 2000, 35–38).

This older cohort, especially the oldest segment of that cohort, has been the beneficiary of federally funded programs from the GI Bill to Medicare. It is important to remember that these highly elaborate institutional forms appeared only in their lifetime; this is the cohort most wedded to those institutions. Later cohorts are much more skeptical that the institutions will remain intact to benefit them in the future. At the same time Medicare appeared, there was a shift in American medical philosophy. The routinization of medical treatments that could extend life led to expectations of longevity. "Dying at age seventy-one or eighty-one is simply unacceptable because one can employ the tools of the clinic to restore health and stave off death." The expectation, at least by middle-class Americans, is that procedures, such as kidney transplants, are a right to be paid for by Medicare (Kaufman, Russ, and Shim 2006, 84). Medicare is not one undifferentiated bureaucratic service, but a complex payment system that includes postre-tirement insurance benefits and low-income Medicaid (Medi-Cal in California); it has become increasingly complex and expensive. New policies, such as supplemental insurance designed to augment Medicare, are costly. Rising drug costs account for most of this increase (Johnson 2006, iii–iv). The advent of **Medicare Part D** in 2006, designed to subsidize the costs of prescription pharmaceuticals, did nothing to simplify the procedure.

In California, 72 percent of large and middle-size firms reported that they provided some prescription drug coverage for retirees (Sauer 2007, 3). The exact nature of that coverage is a vital detail. Coverage for spouses is much more problematic. The Byzantine nature of coverage from multiple sources is only compounded when new elements are added to the bureaucracy. Santa Clara County providers and seniors were asked whether they understood Medicare Part D. This study revealed massive confusion, especially among those least able to cope with the changes, the fiscally and cognitively challenged. One of their participants told them, "The doctor . . . said, 'If I give you this medicine, it will cost you more money.' So he gave me a generic medication. He said he knows that I cannot pay the high price." She goes on to comment, "I did turn down the medicine when I was very ill. The medicine was $145, and I refused to pay. I went without it. I took Tylenol. I don't think I told the doctor though" (De Natale 2007, 177). The complicated nature of copayments and deductibles creates a gap in coverage, a "donut hole" in which the elderly must pay 100 percent of pharmaceutical costs. Only when the costs become "catastrophic," courting destitution, do supplementary benefits begin again. Additional insurance plans for coverage during this hiatus command the most expensive premiums. Navigating this pastiche of plans directs even more of the fixed income of the elderly to health care.

Barbara and Andrew, Still Working, Still Busy

Upon reaching their sixties, workers find retirement is in flux, with no final exit; people move in and out of work. Increasingly, multiple generations of kin are in the workforce, "with all the stresses, joys, responsibilities, and resources such ties entail" (Moen and Roehling 2005, 131–41). Financial security is by no means guaranteed: Social Security is in precarious condition (see Hacker 2008, 128–32). As for private pensions, the situation is even more critical. Twenty-five years ago, 80 percent of the large and medium-size firms offered defined benefits plans in the United States; now fewer than a third do (Hacker 2008, 112).

The life staging of the end of work, of retirement and reduced productivity, permeates the way we talk about our bodies. In his study of veterans Ferzacca (2000, 36–37) was told by the men in the clinic he observed, "Your body is still making insulin, but your body doesn't work well anymore." The pancreas, for these men, was "in retirement." Reminiscent of Hippocratic traditional medicine, there is a form of "humoral biology" in which these retirees link health to productivity. The self-discipline that comes with chronic disease management is somehow at odds with the old idea of retirement as a time of play. In the last stage of work life, taking care of your own body become the "work" of retirement.

Retirement itself is a problematic concept. Not only does retirement depend on a work stage model that has not been intact for decades, but more people are feeling motivated—or experiencing the necessity—to continue working at later ages (Moen and Roehling 2005, 143; Benko and Weisberg 2007, 185). Pension plans no longer provide a guarantee of a secure retirement. Some 63 percent of such pension plans have firm caps on retiree health benefits (Galvin and Delbanco 2006, 1549–50). In California, 51 percent of companies offer defined-benefit pensions (Sauer 2007, 3). When planning for retirement, Americans procrastinate, unwittingly invest in unstable stocks, and get laid off. Given their longevity, such alternatives as 401K plans are not enough to sustain them for the remainder of their lives. Among Americans born from 1931 to 1941, nearly a third have lost half of their wealth—mostly financial assets related to 401K accounts—during the decade from 1992 to 2002 (Hacker 2008, 113–28). The loss of this wealth is forcing retirees back into the job market. While companies declare that they value the skills of retirees, and in California 90 percent of the employers said they would like to retain such employees, the conditions of continued employment are not inviting. Working in retirement can mean employment with reduced pay and responsibilities, shortened schedules, and part-time work with no benefits. Even so, nearly 80 percent of the Californian cohort born after World War II expect to work in retirement (Sauer 2007, 1–5).

Barbara is in her mid-seventies, well past the traditional age for retirement. She has worked all her life, in the space industry in Florida and the personal computer world of Silicon Valley. She enjoys being at the creative center of the technologies that are shaping the world. Barbara has had a heart bypass, but her mother lived until ninety, and she "wouldn't be surprised if I lived to eighty." She works in the administration of a large computer company and cannot really afford to stop working. Her taxes and rent alone are more than her social security income. Her IRA would be enough to live at "the poverty-level for a few years."

Andrew Boland is relatively well educated in navigating his medical coverage, a complex morass that reflects the changes of his former employers' mergers and acquisitions, as well as his transition into retirement. Even though Andrew would be counted among the privileged, his work history demonstrates how the larger structures of corporate churn complicate his retirement. He is seventy-seven and lives with his wife in a moderately prosperous middle-class neighborhood. He had worked in telecommunications all his life. When he began his career, he delivered telegrams. His company changed as the telecommunications sector was revolutionized, and his jobs changed with it. He spent thirty-five years in that company, retired, and began to work at a start-up. Then he worked for another company, which was bought by his original telecommunications employer. That corporate merger was a problem, since he could not work for the same company that was already giving him a pension! Then the company was sold again. Andrew remembers, "Then they had us for about another two years, and they sold us again. Then I was there for another two years, three years, and they sold us, and then another three years and they sold me again. So I kept getting sold all the time along the way there."

He finally retired voluntarily at seventy-two. Andrew spends a significant part of his time caring for himself. He juggles many overlapping conditions: cardiovascular disease, angina, hypertension, osteoporosis, arthritis, allergies, acid reflux, and an enlarged prostate. For these conditions he has had two angioplasty surgeries and a quadruple bypass, and he wears a pacemaker. Andrew gets his prescription medications from the **AARP** pharmacy. He belonged to an HMO, but it was reorganizing and he would have had to change physicians to remain with it. He didn't want that, so he started shopping for another plan. He had a few too many pre-existing conditions for most, and finally "gave up" and adopted a "senior" plan. It supplements Medicare, but not for medication. That means $300 or $400 flies out of his pocket every month. Andrew is well pensioned, possesses high-value property, and has educated himself about his options. However, it would take only a tiny shift in his profile of medication to increase his out-of-pocket expenses to thousands a month; then his financial security would disappear.

After Andrew retired completely he redirected his efforts, noting, "It was difficult. I still woke up early in the morning there for a few months and got ready to go to work. But other than that, I got over it. I don't miss work much. I miss the people; I like the people." He still keeps in touch with those people, meeting them around four times a month. Although Andrew does not get the monthly paycheck, he still engages in the discipline of work, for his community and on himself. He volunteers, providing job-training for the "homeless and underprivileged."

Jean, Leah, and Meg, Taking Care, Giving Back

The productivity of the emerging elderly is not limited to paid work. Theodore Roszak critiques the idea of "productive aging," saying that it is a problematic economic metaphor that does not adequately embrace the desire to be well and to do good (Roszak 2001, 35, 134). A person can want to help society through volunteering or choosing a wholly different service-oriented career—perhaps in health or education. Leah worked twenty years at her national laboratory; each day seemed a grind under her micromanaging administrator. At fifty-five, Leah could easily retire. However, she is going back to the university, taking advantage of a 90 percent tuition reimbursement program. She wants to have a "value somewhere," so she is retraining herself for human services work, saying, "I need to have a purpose." While her friends talk about going on a cruise or moving to the Sierras when they retire, Leah is inspired by a woman she met who worked with the elderly. Maybe a master's in gerontology is in her future? She hopes she can thrive financially "by doing good."

Among Christians, there is a very specific cultural narrative of "doing good" as one ages. In this Christian life stage the elder years are an opportunity to do everyday ministry (Miriam Lueck, Institute for the Future, personal communication). Meg, who suffers from debilitating fibromyalgia, still struggles to fulfill this dream. Meg yearns "to do some kind of ministry. I take every opportunity that I have to be a blessing to someone else as my day goes along, whether that's on the phone or whenever I am in contact with a person—no matter where I am. If I can make their day better, I take that. That's my ministry. I glom onto that opportunity to just be able to bless somebody because I'm starving to do it!" This vision of giving back and doing good is the resurrection of the idealistic values of this generation's youth, values blunted by pragmatic realities but still striving to be expressed. However, such visions do not always mesh with realities. Meg does find it difficult to do her ministry because she spends nearly every waking moment taking care of her own chronic condition—balancing research on her condition, stretching, and self-medication with "motion economy." She has the everyday objects in her environment laid out just so, minimizing the effort needed to navigate her world as she experiences crushing exhaustion. Self-care consumes her time and energy and makes her ideal of late-life-stage ministry less realizable.

Americans born just before and after World War II face an intractable challenge. They are aging into chronic problems that require more direct and intense care, just as they must also juggle the care of parents, spouses, and children. Parents are living longer and their children may be younger, because they gave birth late in life. Yet, in an era of declining medical benefits, where will the resources to provide that care come from? Those still in the workforce need to be employed to retain their work-based insurance benefits. If the problems that require care are severe enough, simply having benefits may not be enough. These older workers must navigate workplace and public policies that do not lend themselves to taking time to deliver care, especially when the cost of living is high and the moral value of work is extreme, in places such as Silicon Valley. Care takes resources, and the age group born after World War II faces the largest rich-poor gap of any American cohort. They generated wealth by working, investing, and creating, but not saving. They have invested time, labor, and money in industries that have disappeared as new technologies replaced them, forcing this age group to reinvent themselves. Some in this age cohort have been able to keep their assets from evaporating, and they will have resources to draw upon for future health care. In sharp contrast, others in that generation have little wealth left (see Vian 2007, 2). In the Silicon Valley region, these class distinctions overlap with "racial" inequalities. Ethnic populations in this age cohort are expected to experience increased health disparities as they age into dependence upon saving and real wealth (Health Research for Action 2007, 81).

Van, Larry Jay, and Emma, Chutes and Ladders

The children's board game Chutes and Ladders suggests a metaphor for the dilemma that faces the elders who are outside the dubious safety zone of job-based health care. In this game of chance, players proceed along a path complicated by a series of ladders and chutes. The ladders allow a player to jump ahead; the chutes send the player significantly backward. Originally a game from India, *moksha-patamu*, play was designed to illustrate karma, demonstrating the consequences of behaving virtuously or evilly. Players find themselves ascending or descending quickly as they land on squares of virtue or evil. British Victorians adapted the structure and morality of the game. Americans softened the moral messages—drawings on the board "good" and "bad" childhood actions—but in this version there are also more ladders to increase the chances of winning (Masters 1997). In my analytical imagination, I can see that "aging well" means having the resources and the circumstances to climb the ladders, to do all the right things by drawing on biomedical and alternative practices to enhance well-being. Taking medications correctly is a ladder, as is access to nutritious food. Winning is made more likely by having a well-structured net-work of support. Needing to care for others can be a dramatic chute, as is the absence of adequate resources. For those who take care of themselves or others, reaching a ladder barely makes up for falling down a chute. Self-sac-rifice can be a chute, while finding supportive others to help or discovering the disciplined morality of self-care may constitute a ladder. This game is played for the highest stakes imaginable—to be a good and healthy per-son.

For the oldest cohort, at least the ones that remain in the Silicon Valley region, the work to be done is the work of caring for their own—and often their spouse's—health. Those who can afford to stay and use medical care available in the region have a significantly different experience from those who live at the margin. Access and adherence are the problems that plague the retired and underemployed elders of the region.

Van Strauss is seventy-three years old, retired from his office work in the insurance industry. Van works on himself now. His house is cluttered, and there are paths through the front room to the couch, and through the hallway to the kitchen, bathroom, and bedroom. His wife's eighty-nine-year-old mother lives with them and is ailing; this is a significant chute. They keep a few basic foodstuffs in the house but eat out 90 percent of the time. Van has the local restaurants mapped out for diabetes-friendly menus and portions. He gets tips from his buddies in his Weight Watchers group. He is so glad that the group has changed over the years. It had been domi-nated by women, who always wanted to *talk* about their weight when they stepped on the scales. Now there are enough men to deflect conversation away from child-rearing to interesting topics, such as "guns and cars, not just keeping the house business."

Van knows the genetic dice are loaded against him. His great uncle had diabetes, but he managed it and lived well into his nineties. His cousin, on the other hand, didn't want to manage it and so lost both his feet. "Then he decided to die, so he died." Van used to work on a farm, and weight was not an issue. Serving in the armed forces he "smoked and smoked and smoked" but kept the weight off. When he returned to the farm he paced himself, doling out a cigarette at the end of each plowed row. One day he just got fed up with that and quit, and the weight started to come on. When he moved to Northern California and took a desk job, the pounds began to creep up: 200, 210, 225, 240, and finally 300. At thirty-five years of age his toes were getting numb and he was diagnosed with diabetes, dropping him down a major chute. Then the struggle began. Juggling a job, two children, and health management, he would get his weight down, only to watch it climb again. Two bouts with colon cancer and a cornea transplant marked his retirement. So he marshaled his resources and enacted a plan of action.

Van's goals are modest, but clear. He hovers around his ideal weight of 190 pounds, walking ten to fifteen miles a week. Van wants to shed at least two more pills from his daily regimen of six: Lipitor, Glucophase, Digitek, over-the-counter baby aspirin, multivitamins, and glucosamine "for old people." In his work he had used a computer and then became a serious home user in the 1980s, experimenting with Gopher, the precursor of the worldwide web, along with being a ham radio operator. Van today surfs the web for health information, especially from his health insurer's website. He trusts them to be straight with him. This website emphasizes the value of sustained moderate exercise, something within Van's reach. He connects his glucometer to the computer and graphs his blood glucose. He sees his computer, meter, books, doctor, and telephone as "all interrelated." He has his information pathways mapped out.

Van has also mapped out his physical world. He took the car, and drove around his neighborhood, creating walk routes in one-mile increments. Along with mall walks, these forays are the backbone of his exercise practice. He jokes that even if he uses a wheelchair, he can do the mall walks into his nineties. His world is filled with numeric metrics that he uses to navigate his health. He contemplates working harder and getting his weight down another twenty pounds, possibly freeing himself from medication, but "that's too much work. I'll just stick to pills." So he creates sustainable daily personal practices, augmented by the structures of biomedicine, health insurance, and Medicare. He has been able to take advantage of his personal game's ladders.

At the other end of the income spectrum, Larry Jay is much younger than Van, but has had a much different pathway through his chutes and ladders. Larry is African-American and "lives" in the East Bay, although since he lives in his vehicle it is difficult to affix an exact location to his residence. When he was in his thirties, Larry, like Van, worked in the fields and planted his own garden. As a young man, Larry would "get up every morning, tend to the chickens, the cows, and the horses, feed the pigs. You're exercising. You're doing this; you're doing that—working the fields."

When he moved to the city, Larry encountered chute after chute. As an urban worker, he polished and waxed cars. Larry remembers, "We never wore masks. That could have also had some effect on my system, my lungs." He moved to the city, and began eating processed food. Larry considers, "They process a whole lot of stuff to prolong it, and that goes right into your system." Ten years later they will tell you that "they had to pull it off the shelf . . . and they've already made ten million dollars off of it." Larry provides social commentary, "Most poor black folks have to cook anyway. But still, you're getting cheap bread, cheap chicken with all that fat on it, the meat is cheap, the stuff you used to throw away you're eating nowadays. We're ruining our bodies that way, too. To eat the right kind of food is expensive. You want to go to one of those places that has organic health food, what do you get for three bucks? What do you get for food stamps?" He gained weight and started having a series of injuries: shoulder, hip, back, leg, and ankle. But "I ignored all that." To recommend exercise to Larry is unrealistic. He points out, "You go [somewhere] to work out: it costs money. You don't want to run around your neighborhood because you're afraid of getting mugged." His emphysema and coronary artery disease cannot be "cured," only managed. He wants to give up smoking, "but living in my car, being homeless, worrying about this, worrying about that . . . paying taxes, paying bills, the insurance, you know what I mean? . . . So I'm worried about this and I'm worried about that, see what I'm saying? It's difficult." He has problems with hemorrhoids, and attributes it to not having enough fiber or protein in his diet. When he has a bout of arthritis, using a mechanistic folk remedy he puts WD-40, a mineral spirit solvent, on his joints and wraps it with an ACE elastic bandage.

Larry works off and on in an auto shop, but observes, "Each time I do the work thing, I end up in the hospital." He has emphysema and asthma, coronary artery disease, and hypertension, conditions that worsen when he details cars. In this list of ailments, he is not too different from the others you have met in this chapter. However, most of his medical care comes in emergency room visits. He tracks his medical record as best he can, saying, "Every visit, I go to the emergency room. They give you a whole thing of what's wrong with you—your medical conditions and all that. I throw these in my car. . . . They get this print-out and give it to you. They tell you what to look for." This printout shows the range for normal breathing, and cites what conditions flow from which problem: "Emphysema causes this problem. High-blood pressure causes this problem." Larry Jay's chutes are all too evident. The geography of risk works against him. His lack of a stable place to live and work undermines his ability to track his care, let alone manage his chronic conditions. While he is told to exercise in his neighborhood, he perceives it to be too dangerous. If he were to park his car—that is, his home—in better neighborhoods, he would not be welcome.

It is inscribed on the bodies of the elderly who has money and who does not. Income inequality differentially exposes people—especially those over sixty-five—to stressors, increasing the risk of poor health (Pearlin et al. 2005). Emma is pushing seventy; she is tiny, a bit wizened, with the raspy voice that comes from a lifetime of smoking cigarettes. She and her husband live in a duplex; her adult son lives in the house where she raised her four children. Her husband, seven years her junior, was laid off at age fifty-eight in one of the busts in the Silicon Valley economy. He tried retraining in a health field—surely there is always work in health care—but remains unemployed. Emma was laid off at fifty-nine and did not even bother to look for work. Her husband's retirement income is $312 dollars a month. Their premium for COBRA, a publicly mandated health plan that allows temporary continuation of group health coverage after job loss, is $400. They are living off the rental incomes of the houses she and her husband owned, perhaps their primary ladder in a board full of chutes. "Otherwise we would have to be leaving this area like everybody else is doing. We'd be in the same boat with the rest of them!"

Emma has had a very hard time. Her daughter died of an accidental overdose. Emma herself had a heart attack; she had a cardiovascular stent surgically implanted. Emma suffered kidney failure and went on dialysis. She had full medical coverage when her husband was working. Now she has only Medicare, because her old insurance company refused to work with Medicare at all. She, however, needed something that would pay the bulk of the expenses of her new conditions. Under her old insurance, she would have had to pay $75 each week for dialysis. Medicare, with supplements, pays the whole amount. "Thank God!" Emma comments. She did not find her way through the morass of plans alone, but with the help of her "ladies at Bingo." Emma's husband uses the Veterans Hospital; while his copayment is tiny, it is keenly felt on their limited income. Larry Jay's and Emma Arnold's series of "chutes" illustrate the structural failures of health care delivery in the San Francisco Bay area. As these stories show, for those at risk there are far more chutes than ladders in real life, making it harder to "win." Silicon Valley is a region with a profound gap between those with high-technology-generated wealth and those who occupy the lower echelons of the economy. For this latter group, disparities often reflect an old American divide—race.

Diverse Disparities

California's inequalities are often described in racialized terms, and there is demonstrable evidence that social hierarchy follows the shifting categories of racial and ethnic identity. However, in terms of health, it is important to remember that one underlying issue for health inequality is the underlying distribution of resources—that is, the differences in class (Farmer 2005, 45). To understand this inequality, we need to review the complex stories of California's and Silicon Valley's economic and symbolically understood diversity.

The contradictions in California's mixture of ethnic and social diversity are evident in its history. In the nineteenth century the Gold Rush, the growth of agriculture in the state, and industrial development created a magnet in California, pulling immigrants from diverse parts of the world. From raisins to railroads, there was work to be had. Critical masses came from specific sites, so that Chinese, Japanese, East Indian, Pilipino, and ever-renewable Mexican workers could form distinct communities. African-American pioneers, Latino *Californios,* and Native Americans, although not immigrants per se, formed substantial populations, often under conditions of extreme stress (Starr 2005, 98–100, 94–95).

The sheer scale of difference created a climate of acceptance, except when it fostered fear and loathing. The 1913 Alien Land Act and earlier legislative acts and court decisions aimed at containing Asians underscored the sentiment of intolerance that sat side by side with attitudes of permissiveness (ibid., 223). Californians both needed, and resented, the presence of diverse peoples. In a form of ethnic tectonics, slowly moving the social order, immigrants come into the labor sector at the bottom of the hierarchy. In a cultural subduction, past migrants would be pushed up the social scale as new peoples migrated in, occupying the lowest sectors. This generations-long migratory pattern is so historically stable it is referred to as "the California pattern," and it has swept ethnic group after group into the cultural mix.

High-technology Asian immigrants in the last two decades of the twentieth century have broken out of the California pattern, but they still encounter a glass ceiling, a barrier to management and entrepreneurship that threatened to turn them into technological "coolies." Only ethnic networking and the establishment of rival and complementary high-technology centers abroad provided the leverage for these South and East Asian immigrants to continue to thrive (Shih 2006; Wong 2006; Varma 2002). Diverse and less formally educated people trapped in the old "California pattern" do not fare so well.

Historians Pitti and Matthews document the inequalities directed at minorities, immigrants, and working-class women who composed the nonelite labor force canning peaches, and staffing the tilt-up fabrication plants that made the personal computer revolution real (Matthews 2003; Pitti 2003). Ethnographer Christian Zlolniski tracks the efforts of undocumented workers from Mexico and Central America who populated the informal economy through the booms and busts of the 1980s and 1990s. They struggled to establish unions, especially to win living wages and health benefits, at a time when such service work was increasingly being

contracted out to temporary employment centers, resistant to labor organization. The mobilization led to increased activism in Latino communities
around education, community development, and political mobilization,
but the region did not embrace unionism (Zlolniski 2003; Zlolniski 2006).
Labor activist Raj Jayadev estimates that minorities make up most of the 20
percent of Silicon Valley's labor force that work under "sweatshop" conditions (Helweg 2004, 62).

In spite of a reputation for natural conservation and ever-expanding
protected open spaces—some 150,000 acres by 2008—other environmental
indicators tell a different story about the region (Henton et al. 2008). The
distribution of environmental toxins demonstrates the persistence of structural inequalities. High-technology industries can be considered clean only
in contrast with Dickensian London or one of Upton Sinclair's industrial
dystopias. Pollutants, particularly from the era of semiconductor production, lurk unseen. Silicon Valley boasts twenty-nine Superfund sites, specific locations designated for federal oversight when hazardous waste or
industrial toxins pose a risk to public health in the absence of a party that
can responsibly attend to manage the clean-up.

The high churn rate for companies makes locating responsible par-
ties even more problematic in Silicon Valley. A full half of the companies
founded in 1982 no longer existed by 2002 (Public Policy Institute of California 2004). Historically working-class areas, such as Mountain View,
Sunnyvale, Santa Clara, and South San Jose, contain the bulk of the sites.
Alviso, an overwhelmingly working-class Latino community near the Bay's
sewage processing and salt flats, is classified as a Superfund site, largely
contaminated with asbestos (Park and Pellow 2004; Pellow and Park 2002).
The year 1981 marked a seminal event when it was discovered that approximately 14,000 gallons of trichloroethane (TCA), a solvent used to remove
grease from manufactured circuit boards, had been leaking into the drinking water for South San Jose (Park and Pellow 2004, 215). In the 1990s, Toxic
Release Inventory data for air pollutants correlated directly to neighborhoods with more Latinos. The more low-income Latinos in a region, the
greater the likelihood that a Toxic Release Inventory site would reside there
(ibid., 217).

Although highly contested, a series of epidemiological studies suggest that electronics production workers in Silicon Valley had three times the rate of occupationally related illness compared with other basic industries. These illnesses include miscarriages, birth defects, and brain, lung, and breast cancers (ibid., 218). One well-known case of occupational illness began in 1998. IBM workers, or their survivors, demonstrated a cancer cluster in South San Jose. Plaintiffs contended that exposure to acetone, benzene, and trichloroethane were directly linked to workers' cancers. They asserted—based on the testimony of a longtime IBM chemist—that the company had been alerted to the danger but did nothing. Jurisprudent drama ensued as judge, jury, and the corporate defendant disagreed. Ultimately, the jury vindicated IBM, and the judge sent the cases to a mediator for settlement out of court by 2004 (Poletti 2004).

This litany of environmental problems underscores the hidden **structural violence** built into the very economic development that distinguishes the region, in spite of the relative absence of overt conflict between socioeconomic classes and groups. In order to understand the relationship between health and work, the structural obstacles to equal well-being must be acknowledged. The distribution of health care and health problems in the region bears this out. Insurance rates vary by ethnicity and class. While 96 percent of English speakers have health insurance—primarily through employer-based coverage—rates for Vietnamese and for Spanish speakers have declined since 2001 to roughly seven in every ten people (Henton et al. 2008, 30). Some 93 percent of Euro-Americans in Santa Clara County are covered, while only 68 percent of Latinos cobble together third-party payments (Fenstersheib 2007, 7). In Silicon Valley the risk for low-income workers intensified as the San Jose Medical Center closed in 2004 and the Regional Medical Center terminated Medi-Cal contracts that had provided an additional safety net (see Photograph 11). In 2005, 119,000 people had no usual place to go to receive care (Auerhahn et al. 2007, 11, 31).

Immigrants are much less likely to be insured (Health Research for Action 2007, 50). Women, too, are more vulnerable. Nearly 11 percent of the men in 2006 reported they lacked health insurance, but nearly 24 percent of women stated they lacked this asset (Health Research for Action 2007,

30). The distribution of health insurance maps directly onto income; in 2005, some 99 percent of the top twentieth percentile had coverage, while only 79 percent of the bottom twentieth had insurance (Henton et al. 2005, 21). About one-quarter of uninsured Santa Clara County residents reported that they could not afford the premiums, and another third had lost or changed jobs, underscoring the systemic link between employment and access to biomedical care (Health Research for Action 2007, 30). The retired and near-retired workers of Silicon Valley differ in both obvious and subtle ways. Clearly, socioeconomic stability, at a time in the life course when economic constancy is a challenge, will dramatically separate the experiences of the wealthy and the poor. This watershed is exaggerated by the high cost of living and the already extant rich-poor divide. The people who are systematically limited in their participation in the workforce—by age, race, or class—do not have job-based health plans and cannot earn the money to afford private insurance. Structural social barriers contribute to failed health through a reduced access to health care, an inability to mobilize healthy behaviors, and a degradation of residential and workplace environments. These structural failures demonstrate the reciprocity between productivity and health. Productive workers are able to be healthier than those who are barred from the bureaucracies and benefits of employment. Healthy people, in the social and physical prime of life, can buffer the impact of the economy more easily than the vulnerable poor and elderly. The intimate linkage between employment and health makes work-centered Silicon Valley a prime site for understanding the embodiment of labor.

6   Tinkering with the Future

And if you dont like the tone
*   of my poems*
You can go jump in a lake.
I have been empowered
*   To lay my hand*
On your shoulder
*   and remind you*
That you are utterly free,
Free as empty space.
—Kerouac 1995, "11th Chorus," 127

Project Well-Being

Work dominates Silicon Valley life, influencing governance, family life, self-management, and self-care. In part, this reflects the close association of the workplace with the structures of health care. Without work, there is no work-based insurance. Such an infrastructure, however, is changing. Contract work, short-tenure employment, high-tech rates in which companies rapidly appear and disappear—all make this association churn problematic in this region. Most important, the shift of responsibility from organization to individual, a key feature of late capitalism, has implications for self-care. Individuals are supposed to be unfettered creative innovators, while managing the mundane details of their pensions and health plans. Workers are responsible for projects and for themselves as projects. Silicon Valley, an early adopter of this corporate philosophy, provides an illustration of the results of such changes. It is one of the key ways in which people, in the guise of workers, *feel* capitalism.

Everyday people have come, by birth or choice, to live in California's greater San Francisco Bay Area, which combines immigration-driven diversity, social creativity, and countercultural activism to create a distinctive health culture. This deep medical diversity provides an array of conceptual and material tools drawing on traditional health practices, innovative syntheses and holistic healing modalities to combine with biomedicine. Medical schools at the University of California, San Francisco, and Stanford, along with a vast halo of both private and nonprofit medical organizations, ensure that biomedicine is amply represented.

Along the northern Californian coast, this regional health culture extends from the Esalen Institute at Big Sur (once home to **Gestalt therapy**'s Fritz Perls) to the vineyards and culinary centers of Napa Valley; it surrounds and includes Silicon Valley. In this mecca of high-technology innovation, a different set of values intersects and complements the Bay Area health culture. There, the counterculture, while still valuing the "natural," prizes technological solutions. In this local culture, it is held that technological efficiency will give people the tools that they need to realize humanity's potential. Being healthy is not merely an end in itself, but a means to augment self-actualization and productivity.

Silicon Valley does not have an undifferentiated *ethos*, experienced the same way by men and women, venture capitalists and janitors, but exists in a complex ecosystem of ways of feeling and acting. This ecosystem is composed of emotions, ideas, practices, and objects that pass through this center of global flows.[1] Some of the facets of that system are a function of people moving, bringing selected pieces of their culture with them into the region. The emotions generated by different kinds of music, from classical Indian compositions to Urban *Tejano* dance music, reflect the region's diversity. Other practices in the ecosystem are hybrid creations, such as the activities associated with contemporary holistic healing. *Habitus*, or durable dispositions, are those behaviors and ideas to which we are culturally sensitized, and shape different practices around eating, moving, and caretaking. Such intricacy contributes to the deep medical diversity experienced there.

The pragmatism of technologists makes it easy for them to navigate deep medical diversity. Their motto could be "Use any tool that works." Insulin pumps and Chinese herbs are used to manage blood glucose; both double lattes and Ginkgo biloba tablets are consumed to enhance concentration. Cognitive tools facilitate working on oneself and include such practices as neurolinguistic reprogramming, management seminars, and behavioral coaching. The burgeoning industry of working on oneself, from EST to half-day workshops on "visioning," complement the daily self-exploration that takes place in cubicles and at dining tables. Clare's Ganesha shrine sits next to her ergonomic desk. John Carter deviates from his family's Irish-American meat and potato diet with "rice and fish" and counts his "health game points" as if it were a video game. Clare and John are doing identity exploration that would seem familiar in principle, if exotic in practice, to their nineteenth-century American Transcendentalist counterparts.

These social processes are experienced differently across the life stages. Work stage, cohort effect, and aging all play a role in defining how health is felt. The classic prework, work, retirement linear stage is unraveling, to be replaced by a more flexible and unpredictable system. The bodies of Silicon Valley must become resilient amid these changes or suffer the consequences. In this book we saw significant differences among the cohorts. Cognitive styles, such as embracing modularity, shifted. Integration with technology is in an inverse relationship with age. Within families, experimentation in networked relationships, deeply diverse medical practices, and processes of self-augmentation spread from one family member to another. These processes are not unique to Silicon Valley, yet the people of the region are early adopters allowing social scientists and policy-makers to see the consequences of feeling capitalism.

In this final chapter, we will explore the implications that Silicon Valley bodies have revealed. One set of inferences is useful to practitioners of anthropology. This case study reinforces the notion that place is analytically essential. The people you have met are not generic bodies, they are Silicon Valley bodies. Embodiment itself is significant in anthropological thinking, breaking down Cartesian categories to re-create a very particular form of holism.

For anthropologists even to see such phenomena means acknowledging the importance of historic and geographic particularities. At the same time, such particularities should not be essentialized or reified. The embodied cultures, the *habitus* of the region, are durable but not enduring. They change. The embodied productivity experienced by the age cohorts born in the 1930s, 1950s, 1970s, or 1990s shows common cultural ground, but they also differ in significant ways. Modular boundaries are eroding among the younger cohorts; modules—whether technological, physical, cultural, or cognitive— are broken into smithereens and the bits are being mixed and matched. Even strong associations, such as the need for actual biological ancestry to claim cultural identity, are becoming less tightly held by the young.

In Silicon Valley aging is associated with reduced productivity and increased disease. It must be managed and resisted using all the tools available. On the one hand, aging is viewed as an unnatural deficiency to be overcome through technological correction. At the same time, nature, as configured by the countercultural ecological and alternative health movements is an ally to be used to "age well." Nature, associated with a nostalgic vision of the past, is benign and a source of healing. Nature is, in this understanding, sustainable. This notion of nature suggests that proper political action entails conserving and using nature more appropriately. It also naturalizes the indigenous and the weak and pulls in concepts of social justice. "Fair trade," "organic," and "sustainable" merge to become one cognitive construct with subtly different facets, however they might compete otherwise. These values become part of a new global cosmopolitanism, similar to that experienced in Indonesia. Young Indonesians have learned to "love nature," and this romantic affect is an integral part of a cosmopolitan global identity (Tsing 2005, 122–27). Similarly, the trust, affection, and reverence given to nature in the practices of the Bay Area's deep medical diversity are **immanent**, suggesting that the spiritual permeates the biological. The sanctity given the body would be more familiar to Transcendental philosopher poet Ralph Waldo Emerson than mind-body dualist René Descartes.

New harmonics of cultural experience are created when those differences are coexperienced in classrooms, around workplace water coolers, in restaurants and parks. When a ten-year-old experiences a Vietnamese Buddhist playmate's vegetarian dinner, it changes the way she understands, imitates, and embodies elder sister's vegan Berkeley roommates. The purchase of a "green" Sigg bottle—an aluminum container meant to replace disposable plastic water bottles—evolved from a larger transcendental reverence for nature. The romantic "oriental gaze" of transcendentalism shapes how San Jose's Japanese Friendship Garden, rooted in the historic reality of East Asian immigration, is rendered aesthetic. The values of the ecological movement, rooted in historic specificity of the Bay Area counterculture, interact with those of the many diverse ancestral cultures.

Finally, we need to look at the implications of the social experiments that have taken place in Silicon Valley. Productivity is intimately linked with health; both productivity and well-being have become the responsibilities of the workers themselves. In an era of employee-centered health care, the *gaze* of the employer has intensified and broadened to include more of life, even though the *responsibility* rests more firmly on the individual. More workers will employ the tools of deep medical diversity, expecting a range of health care options that is not being included in any statistically validated formulary or traditional human resources scheme. These practices of deep medical diversity will shape the policies of public and private organizations. Repeatedly, regional public health organizations note that health care in the region must acknowledge ethnic and ancestral diversity (Health Research for Action 2007).

Pragmatic Experimentation

The drive for experimentation is a subtle and revolutionary manifestation of twentieth-century transcendental ethics. To work on ones *self* requires setting aside fixed cultural modes. Experimentation is valued in the San Francisco Bay Area and Silicon Valley in particular. Music, politics, sexuality, relationships, technologies, and foods were all subject to playful trial and error. Silicon Valley became known for creating disruptive technologies—approaches designed to introduce whole new concepts and ways of solving problems, not just incremental adjustments to existing patterns. The counterculture tends to be treated as one undifferentiated movement, but there were differences between the new left and Stewart Brand's new communalists, who intended to redesign their relationship to the world through psychedelic experimentation, cross-cultural exploration, and technological augmentation. These new communalists "embraced technocentric optimism, the information theories, and the collaborative work style of the research world" (Turner 2006, 240).

Experimentation over the last few decades was social, as well as technological. The replacement of vertically integrated companies by decentralized networked organizations became the region's critical advantage. Globally linked networks of companies, workers, and capital reshaped the way work was done in distributed teams (see Saxenian 2006). In addition, networked workers were also networked families, who strategically used relationships to access resources and to create personal meaning (Darrah, Freeman, and English-Lueck 2007).

Pragmatism, efficiency, productivity, augmentation—these are the values that emerged from an *ethos* of experimentation, and in turn reinforced it. As soon as the technological framework switched, from replacing humans with artificial intelligence to enhancing them through augmentation, the potential applications for self-experimentation were greatly expanded. Technologies made possible the extension of human cognition, memory, and communication, and provided a new set of cultural metaphors for self-actualization. Tinkering with oneself took on a new meaning. Technology granted widespread access to the health information sphere, in its many biomedical and alternative forms, facilitating deep medical diversity on laptops across the region. If I want to know where I could find Natragest, wild yam progesterone cream, to manage my menopausal symptoms, Google can provide retail options far and near—as well as revealing the best prices, copious reviews, and testimonials. Communities of women experiencing menopause have created blogs, online-hosted groups, and web-based real-time meet-up groups. As *Brand's CoEvolution Quarterly* postulated thirty years ago, the technology serves as a tool not only to build new communities but also to host the communities themselves (Turner 2006, 125–26). The augmentation technologies include not only corrective and restorative prosthetic devices but information and communication tools as well. Artifacts may even include pharmaceuticals, foods, drinks, nutraceuticals, and physical practices. Yoga mats, fair trade coffees, and latte machines are part of the *materia medica* for being productively augmented and morally good.

The practices of neurolinguistic programming stress the specifics of internal linguistic thought to restructure how life is experienced. An injured leg is not a *bad* leg. Practices that support optimism, in the form of repeated affirmations, help the person keep a positive outlook and experience more energy. Prayer and meditation are somaticized, linked to particular postures and places, sites of heightened awareness. Alternative medications and practices, herbal concoctions, and acupuncture are expected to have broadly encompassing impacts on physical sensation, emotional resonance, and a greater openness to spirit.

Restaging

The divisions between age-based life stages are becoming curiously blurred; the different experiences people have across the lifespan, as embodied workers, are becoming less certain. The "lockstep career path" that so organized the life of the American worker in the middle decades of the twentieth century has come to have less meaning (Moen and Roehling 2005). The work ladder is now more of a lattice, with people moving in and out of work jobs and companies throughout their lives (Benko and Weisberg 2007; Moen and Roehling 2005). The youngest cohorts concentrate on preparing themselves for a lifetime of flexible employment. The youngest cohort is native to many of the changes in the region. They are comfortable with digital technologies and expect constant employment reinvention. These young people know only deep medical diversity and deep diversity and so take it as *natural*. Paid work dominates the rhythms and options of people in their late twenties through their sixties. Some form of work restructuring, including redefining their contribution to community engagement, will happen to people as they age. The cohort born after World War II may have helped to create many of these social changes, but they are not native to them. The older the cohort, the more alien these transformations may seem to them.

Education is no longer confined to the young or productive work to adulthood. Education is cast as workforce preparation and enhancement, and individuals may need to retool themselves many times in the course of a career. In Silicon Valley, industry has a significant impact on the way this training is done (English-Lueck 2002). Internships and learning academies bring work ever closer to the curriculum. When adults work at home, young people are drawn into their work practices, as either observers or participants. Sonya and Hettie Schwarz learned their work ethic by participating in their parents' conversations at the family's dinner table.

The period of adult work may be unstable as life events interfere with the ideal career ladder. Parenthood, caretaking, job loss, and career switching all make the old linear path problematic. People step on and off their career paths as life and the economy permit. As we saw with Emma in the last chapter, stepping permanently off that path is also tricky. Retirement may mean career retooling, scaling down, expanding volunteer "work," and working on oneself and others as a caretaker. It rarely means unending leisure in Silicon Valley.

Health culture, especially as it relates to food, exercise, and identity, is also changing. The children of Silicon Valley are native to digitalized deep diversity. They are comfortable with information immersion, surfing multiple contexts and experimenting with new foods, friends, and world views. The younger cohorts are not homogenous, and vary in their access to technologies and cultural commitment to their parents' health practices. They have grown up with their own identities in flux, and in coping with the multiple practices manifested in neighbors and classmates. This third wave has been reared with the San Francisco Bay Area health culture all around them; vegan, tattooed Goths sit alongside Indo-American Desi Bollywood dance aficionados in the region's high school classes. For them, the modularity of American culture, so typical of twentieth-century America, is more fragmented. Modules are made up of different sampled bits, and are subject to "mash-up," what social scientists would call bricolage—a mosaic assembled from available cultural materials. Elements of media, music, movement, philosophy, or cuisine can be mixed, modified, and customized in combinations that suit the tastes of the individual and fit in with the individual's social network of friends, family, and coworkers. They are far less bound to keeping the cultural integrity of the modules.

Exit Descartes, Enter Emerson

There is a continuum, from the most elderly to the youngest cohort, in which increasing comfort with deep medical diversity and deep diversity makes itself manifest in how the mind and body are viewed. In contrast to the third wave, in those people in their fifties and sixties, with their teen and twenty-year-old children and grandchildren, we see the dramatic change that has occurred in the conceptualization of the embodied self.

The oldest cohort appears content with biomedicine itself, if not with its system of delivery and payment. Ben Jensen, Van Strauss, Andrew Boland, and others of their age group live comfortably in their modules of mind, body, and spirit—and tuck each practice tidily into its appropriate compartment. The older the person—at least for those born in the United States—the more the modular foundational schema are intact. Scientific medicine is rooted in Cartesian dualism (Goldstein 1999, 15). The ethnopsychology of dominant "Western" European, American, and Antipodean societies practices a "deep interiorization of self" that reifies its separation (Kleinman and Kleinman 2007, 470). Psychologists and psychiatrists tend the mind, doctors the body, and priests and rabbis the spirit. The cognitive landscape of the elderly more clearly separates the person's mind and body.

The most elderly cohorts also lived through the influx of immigrants and the proliferation of alternative strategies, but did not necessarily embrace them. For many, biomedicine had clear orthodoxy over alternative frameworks. Even elderly immigrants, while they would privilege their own home-country's medical system, would not necessarily question the established biomedical system. For many elderly, challenging the health care delivery system is not an option to be routinely exercised. In this form of engagement, the Cartesian duality of mind-body and perhaps, spirit, remains defined in ways it is not for the younger cohorts of Silicon Valley.

However, for the cohort born immediately before and after World War II, there were profound philosophical reasons for experimenting with alternative medical systems as countercultural notions took hold. The health modules inherited from biomedicine break down as the members of the first wave adopt a new language for the body. English-language discourse has a poor vocabulary for integrative non-Cartesian models, but it is adapting. Is *prana* or *qi* mind, body, or spirit? In the original linguistic contexts, this would be a nonsensical question. The increasingly facile translation of quantitative biomedical metrics into mind-body-spirit qualifiers bespeaks a new type of embodied knowledge. Those people who participated in the countercultural movements of self-actualization, religious experimentation, and alternative healing and eating have *learned* to question Cartesian duality, but lack a comfortable vocabulary to express a singular self. They can easily see emotions and spirit as one, but have a much harder time merging ethereal conditions and the material body. These first wave synthesists can imagine how happiness is intrinsic to well-being, but they find it less clear how to enact the spiritual and emotional healing of embodied chronic disease. This dilemma is at the heart of Joan's attempts to find a spiritual path to manage her diabetes.

The way health is measured in biomedicine reinforces and compounds body-mind dualism. Physical states can be measured; weight, triglycerides, potassium, and fasting glucose levels can be quantified. Energy, vitality, zest, fatigue, and pain are evaluative states that lack tangible metrics. These feelings are much more ephemeral, but no less valid to people trying to rethink Cartesian duality. The first wave cohort continues to experiment in countercultural activities, and struggles to translate one system of accounting to the other. They create and recast tools to help them. Yoga and *qigong* are physical activities that turn attention inward to subjective states.

This knowledge is based not on biomedical, statistical inferences but on an integrated experiential intuition. This does not mean that it is not knowledge. Wine connoisseurs have a whole sensuous vocabulary to talk about nose, aftertaste, body, fruit, brilliance, and oakiness. It is difficult to pinpoint those indeterminate qualities, but it is informed knowledge nonetheless. In a similar way, the subjective experiences of an integrated non-Cartesian person reflect a new evaluative vocabulary (see Kuriyama 2007). The first wave cohort revitalized this ineffable approach to food, self-exploration, and a transcendental connection to nature. They are not native to it, as were those younger folk we met in previous chapters for whom Descartes' dualism is increasingly alien. Members of the second and third wave of integrators have continued the epistemological breakdown of the separate modules of mind, body, and spirit. The consequences of deep medical diversity have been partially enacted by the younger adults, who are subject to job-based health insurance, wellness programs, and the consumption of health and beauty products and practices. Their children see themselves in an even more cosmopolitan and all-encompassing marketplace of wellness behaviors. Acting as parents, teachers, and employers, first wave participants may have been seminal in combining practices and experimenting with new healing modalities, but they still find themselves looking for institutional health care solutions.

There are real structural and legal institutional constraints on alternative healing. Rarely, with the exception of osteopathic, chiropractic, and some acupuncture services, are CAM treatments compensated by a third-party insurance payment system. Most of the $47 billion in alternative medicine expenditures is spent out of pocket (Barnes et al. 2004). While prayer may not be costly, provisioning nutraceuticals and making homes "natural and toxin-free" takes resources. This fiscal structure inserts alternative healing into the marketplace and so limits access. Moreover, the licensing structure in California constrains overt practice. Acupuncturists must be trained at approved sites, and naturopaths can be overt providers of care only as long as they don't impinge on the purview of biomedicine. Homeopaths and massage therapists must recast themselves as teachers or healing peers (Baer 2001b, 332; English-Lueck 1990). The health care bureaucracies most used by the elderly tend to exclude complementary and alternative healing. The deep medical diversity of the region drives experimentation with alternative practices. Young people have been enculturated into and experienced the deep medical diversity that integrates mind and body, and adds spirit to the mix. People experiencing deep medical diversity inject spirituality into embodied practices and transform cognitive states into physical sensations. Just as traditional Chinese medicine is based on a separate tradition that was not subject to the logic of Descartes, which would segregate mind (spirit)-body, such duality makes little sense to the youngest cohort who practice alternative and immigrant-based health care. People in their teens and early twenties understand their health status by drawing on diverse explanations—genetics, karma, and active behavioral modification. People socialized in it from a young age—the digital natives—are also born into deep medical diversity, a health culture that combines a dense array of practices drawn from immigrant traditions, alternative health, and biomedicine. They are much less tied to the Cartesian split of mind-body.

Anthropology and the Ghost of Descartes

The foundational framework separating mind and body has influenced the very models by which anthropologists view humanity. Although introductory textbooks consistently refer to anthropology as holistic, within anthropology the ghost of Descartes continues to haunt. We have divided our discipline into specializations that focus on cognition, or linguistically informed symbolic approaches to the human experience. Other forms of anthropology track inequalities of power or epidemiological patterns; their data set is more often material than abstract and ideational. The very division in American anthropology between cultural and physical reifies a presumed mind-body partition.

In the final two decades of the twentieth century, the theoretical positions of postmodernism and poststructuralism drew on humanistic epistemologies that seemingly underscored their differences from concrete empirical anthropological approaches. In interpretive anthropology, hermeneutics is the interpretation of cultural meaning, especially in language, ritual events, and social institutions. Such interpretation favors abstract, symbolic, and intangible evidence and reflects a humanistic approach. Alternative medical beliefs and Silicon Valley company discourses are appropriate subjects for such analyses. Anthropologists using that approach infer abstract insights from the symbolic qualities of behavior or material objects. In contrast, biological, ecological, and epidemiological patterns are extrapolated from the tangible. Public health personnel test animals and people to find particular pathogens. People in Santa Clara County fall prey to the West Nile virus, and are carriers of resistant tuberculosis. Patterns of global agricultural exchange and immigration explain such pathogenic mobility, based on material evidence. Privileging of one form of evidence over another has led to a dual anthropological reality. The cognitively constructed imaginary realm is viewed as distinct from the measurable external physical realm. As Bruno Latour suggests, these assumptions led to the strange invention of the "mind-in-the-vat" that sits "in opposition to outside world" (2007, 179–80).

A subtle Cartesian division is implicit in American anthropological thought. A person's thought and emotions reside in the brain, to be parsed as either a physical process or a symbolic sociolinguistic formulation. Such anthropological theory begins by "denaturalizing" the body—positing that cultural knowledge is constructed about, in, and through material realities, including our organic selves. The concept of *embodiment* deliberately blurs the barriers between material and mental. Social philosophers Charles Taylor and Pierre Bourdieu popularized this experimental thinking. Embodiment suggests that culture is not an abstract floating miasma that somehow percolates into consciousness, but a set of guidelines that are made manifest in practices inscribed in the body. From Latin America to China, medical anthropologists have long been studying systems that are not based on Cartesian duality. Forcing traditional medical epistemologies into models based on separating mind and body has worked poorly. These medical anthropologists realized that embodiment, as a theoretical device, meant that the curious curse of narrative fixation—the increasing abstraction of cultural phenomena—could be removed. Anthropologists could get beyond isolating the products of the brain—abstractions and words—to the *practices* of everyday life. Such ethnographic life is not an abstract text, removed from personal experience, but exists with intense materiality. People do not just *have* bodies as if their consciousness resided elsewhere; they *are* embodied.

The rift between materialist and mentalist anthropologists is healed, however, as they have begun to put the "mind back in the body back in the world" (ibid. 2007, 182). The key to this reconciliation is embodiment. The body is not somehow "natural" in opposition to an artificial cultural construct. Bodies are not *just* natural objects, but they are changed by the experience of cultural actions and imaginings. This synthesis of critical symbolic and empirical physical approaches "opens" the possibility to view human experiences as "subjective and objective, carnal and conscious, observable and legible" (Lock and Farquhar 2007, 11). Luke is not just a diabetic body. He considers himself augmented by the opportunity to monitor and understand himself better. But his understanding is situated in his body; he subjectively links his numbers to his state of being. Experiences are also not *merely* processed through an abstracted consciousness, but that awareness is embodied and in the world.

Phenomenologist Maurice Merleau-Ponty influentially posits that consciousness is "mediated through experienced embodiment." However, he argues his case based on logical premises that are fundamentally universal; he is not concerned with the peculiarities of historic or geographic distinctions. Pierre Bourdieu, on the other hand, explores distinct social realities, making embodiment relevant for anthropological inquiry (ibid., 6–7). Merleau-Ponty considers humanity in a general sense, while Bourdieu's humans were specific to locations: Kabyle men in colonial Algeria and bachelors in southwestern rural France. Bourdieu argues that specific social conditioning creates "durable dispositions" of thought, taste, feeling, and bodily posture; he calls these states *habitus* (Bourdieu 1998, 7; Reed-Danahay 2005, 103; Bourdieu 1977). The embodied dispositions of *habitus* translate the social structures of power and place them in the body. With an awareness of power heightened by the influence of Foucault, *habitus* is not culturewide but specific to class and social position. The embodied cultural experience of the educated French elite is fundamentally different from that of the French peasant. *Habitus* is *ethos*, a concept long used in psychological anthropology, revisited for the highly complex stratified societies of the postcolonial world. The most obvious example from this book comes from Larry Jay, the homeless auto detailer. For Larry, physical activity properly belongs in the field or the shop floor. He disdains "working out." Such activity is elitist, and in his neighborhood, unsafe. He does not experience the compulsion embodied by Joan or Jean to have a daily yoga-based practice in order to feel complete.

In the distinctive health culture explored in this book, new criteria are being added to the array of *habitus*. The introduction of ethnic and organic foods stimulates a new sensibility to freshness, spiciness, and color. "Asian" body postures, softer and suppler, compete with and complement rigid "European" body-builder images. The resulting cultural ergonomics— from Asia and elsewhere—change the way people in the region sit, stand, and move. Yoga becomes part of physical therapy, and German isometric strength-training creeps into Chinese martial arts. Deep medical diversity reflects the blending of anthropological divisions. Immigrant and "traditional" medical beliefs and practices are not separate and distinct from the alternative health movements. Among the new practices in Silicon Valley are ones oriented toward building an individual's resilience in the workplace that is assumed to be polluted, hostile, and unreliable.

Stephen Kunitz (2007), public health historian, suggests that the scientific seekers for the social determinants of health are always searching for the central tendency along a presumed normal curve. Hence they overlook those particulars that actually drive how people experience disease. The specific details of work settings, historical values, geopolitical regions, and governmental credos shape patterns of health and disease. Historical particulars allow anthropologists to see more exactly how this ecosystem of health-related *habitus* works. The San Francisco Bay Area health cultures, and the even more particular Silicon Valley *habitus* of productivity, are not replicated in exactly the same way elsewhere.

However, focusing rigorously on specifics does not mean that we cannot learn about the processes of health embodiment that may be generalized to a wider realm. How do specific communities express their "traditional" health cultures? What are the means by which those not born into those cultures become exposed to particular practices? How do "traditional" and "alternative" practices inform each other? Who are the early adopters of such practices? How do those deep medical pluralities change over time, across cohorts, and in different communities of practice? How do larger forces, such as individuated consumer capitalism, mold the purposes, expressions, and outcomes of deep medical diversity? These questions are generalizable, and the processes revealed overarching, even if the exact answers are particular to a given cultural location.

The undermining of Cartesian approaches, whether by philosophers, anthropologists, or twenty-three-year-olds working at Google, means rethinking how we view "health." As the body is reunited with the socially constructed mind, health itself expands to include beauty, fashion, spirituality, bio-mechanical augmentation, and productivity. Health is not the purview of body mechanics, but a larger set of practices that are distributed across a person's life.

Three Experiments

The implications for care, payment, and policy change when health is viewed as a set of practices. Deep medical diversity, then, becomes interesting to more than public health theorists and anthropologists. Biomedical providers, alternative health practitioners, nonprofit community health workers, human resources specialists, and corporate managers all need to understand what it means to function competently in a deeply diverse medical situation.

The Silicon Valley region's social "laboratories" are running three experiments—*embodied productivity, worker-centered wellness care,* and *deep medical diversity.* These novel practices have different and overlapping meanings for corporations, nonprofit organizations, families, and networks of individuals. Embodied productivity refers to the practices of work as performed by living people who use their bodies to intensify their output. Within Silicon Valley some of their employers, and public and nonprofit partners, are pioneering worker-centered wellness programs that rethink the traditional relationship implicit in employee benefits. These wellness practices are configured around the health cultures that have developed in Silicon Valley, a region deeply diverse. Applied to health, this means that traditional medical beliefs, *materia medica,* and alternative health practices feed back on one another to create a deep medical diversity that intensifies health experimentation. Silicon Valley and San Francisco are also at the forefront of innovative biomedical research and clinical experimentation. In any person's given social network there will be a deeply diverse array of practices, information sources, and evaluative opinions to draw upon to address their health needs.

Embodied Productivity

These stories of Silicon Valley explore the intensification of individuation around work and health. Work is the workers' problem, particularly in the shifting corporate landscape of high-technology and the halo of businesses that service it. Ubiquitous communications technologies mean that even client-based work can be done remotely; such interactions do not need to be face to face. Work, and the compulsion to work, can creep into the rest of life. Individuals are expected to create and modulate their own skill sets, adapting to a constantly changing labor market. Flexible autonomy is not limited to the technological elite, but extends to the creative service sectors that support them. As more work is conceptualized as independent project-based work, individuals must apply management techniques to themselves to get the job done, whether that work is done at home, in the car, in a hotel, or in a designated workspace.

The volatility and intensity of Silicon Valley's economy is a palpable source of health stress. In his Sunnyvale family's story, author Jeff Goodell relates the story of his father, a man who never quite succeeded as Santa Clara County morphed into Silicon Valley. His father graduated from Palo Alto High School in the 1950s, overweight, with dermatological problems, and was eventually diagnosed with Cushing's Syndrome. This disease was caused by an adrenal tumor, and the gland was surgically removed. His son later writes, "The surgery that saved his life also left him invisibly crippled. Without adrenal glands, his body could not produce adrenaline. No wonder he later seemed so maladapted to the world he lived in. Without adrenaline, he literally lacked the fuel that made Silicon Valley go" (Goodell 2000, 42–44).

Workers are also rewarded for being and looking productive. Productivity can be accounted for by measuring and quantifying the product created, but there are other metrics. It is a drama that can be demonstrated qualitatively by the visible appearance of being *better than well*. Hence the need for enhancements—diet Coke, coffee, vitamins, workouts, even prescription drugs. Cosmetic neurology, including hormonal therapy, and "neurochemicals used by healthy people to stimulate productivity" accompany cosmetic alteration to boost or recapture the productivity of youth. The cultural definitions of deficiency, normality, and enhancement are being rewritten. Anthropologist Linda Hogle (2005, 695–96), who investigates **enhancement medicine**, notes, "What distinguishes these techniques is that bodies and selves become the objects of improvement work, unlike previous efforts in modernity to achieve progress through social and political institutions. There are profound effects on sociality and subjectivity." However, when talking about these new states, we emphasize individual choice and agency. We make such feelings seem innate, rather than seeing affect as a "capitalist construction," a by-product of the economic system we have created (Kleinman and Kleinman 2007, 472). Middle-class aesthetics and health disciplines are utterly integrated with "consumer and capitalist culture" (Lock and Farquhar 2007, 491).

Embodied productivity reflects a shift in how businesses think of workers. The creation of a disembodied worker, whose function is production, is fundamental to twentieth-century Taylorized industrial logic. Skills are broken into pieces and distributed so that the entire process of production is maximally efficient. The management of such a process treats workers as disembodied abstractions. Much of the labor history of the twentieth century was an attempt by workers to force recognition of their individual embodied humanity—seeking better and safer work conditions, health, family, and retirement benefits. Innovative knowledge work, in particular, requires an intensity that involves the whole person, not just a bit of abstract thought here, as if the brain were working on its own. Such professional work has largely been treated as an abstract act of "embrained" thought-based or **encoded knowledge**—the kind of symbolic knowledge found in books, manuals, and codes of practice. However, as ethnographers observe the actual work practices, we see that much of the work of the new economy is not really so abstract. Embodied knowledge—practical hands-on problem-solving—is much more tangible and inherently social. Workers, especially obvious in complex diverse teams, use encultured knowledge that emphasizes shared understandings and common metaphors (Williams 2006, 591). Creative work in particular relies on workers being in their bodies in social contexts. People use lateral thinking from games, hobbies, and casual conversations with friends and family to make art, solve problems, and design products. As organizations recognize the validity of putting workers back in their bodies, and back in the world, they must pay attention to the embodied conditions in which they work.

In contemplating cultural futures, it is always problematic to separate out desirable, undesirable, and probable scenarios. Finding ethnographic evidence of how people think about the future is invaluable in sorting out what people intend. This region foreshadows what the future holds for many. As science-fiction writer William Gibson (1999) is often quoted as saying, "The future's already here, it's just not very evenly distributed." Silicon Valley's embodiment of health points to a series of thorny issues that reflect *feeling* capitalism. Disease, measured by a series of quantifiable metrics, is unequally distributed. That health care disparities exist in the United States is hardly news. Unequal access to medical care, the tools needed to change behavior, and the ability to minimize stressors map neatly onto the rich-poor gap. Larry Jay introduced us to his reality in which access to any care but emergency rooms is limited. Fresh produce and daily walks in the neighborhood are not part of his social experience. Just because the *average* life span has increased does not mean there are not significant disparities. Advocates of *better than well*, with access to the tools needed to make that vision plausible, are in sharp contrast to those that, at best, merely manage their disease burden with increasing difficulty. Infrastructural changes in the way risk is apportioned and insured mean that differential access to care is built into the current American system. The notion of individual empowerment with its individuated responsibility is in conflict with the very idea of broadly pooling risk. Those with the ability to mobilize resources feel confident that such tools are universal. That *habitus* feels real to them, but it is an artifact of their point of view. Access to care, good food, emotional well-being, and opportunities for safe exercise are not individual choices, but are subject to structures of power. Structural dilemmas require structural management, and calls for large-scale changes in the American health care "system" are widespread as more and more people are left without a medical safety net. That potential reformation is a work in progress at the end of the first decade of the twenty-first century.

While such a large-scale change constitutes a desirable future, it is not necessarily a probable one. Pragmatically, the American social reality of the next decade will most likely reflect a system of comparable commodified care, with continued experimentation by individuals, networks, and organizations. It is in that experimentation that Silicon Valley's experience can inform policy, both pubic and private.

Meanwhile, social networks are mobilized to provide information and evaluate particular practices regarding health *repair*. However, they are also used to create a repository of wellness practices, increasingly aimed at avoiding the necessity of intensive care. Individuals are seeking therapeutic interventions with the goal of becoming physically sustainable workers. Aging well is a central discourse to this practice. Finally, networks are literally a source of legal and illegal pharmaceuticals, practices, and technologies to become better than well. Devices and pharmaceuticals designed to augment a worker's abilities are shared and promoted within networks. From the earliest days of ingesting LSD to wearing the body monitoring devices used by dedicated bicyclists, networked practices reflect embodied experimentation and adoption.

Whether in tandem with institutional change or outside it, individuals themselves will mobilize their social networks to provide support that is as ubiquitous as their work-home-health environments. Coworkers already solicit help from each other with health advice, nursery school information, and financial advising. Pam Ibarra recalls that her husband's oncologist expected that he would use his coworker network and computer expertise to educate himself about his disease. Coparents, the mothers and fathers of one's children's friends, are asked for employment tips as well as sharing child care. Employers benefit from this networked knowledge.

Ethnographic evidence suggests that people creatively enact networked expertise and resources. Individual workers' information networks extend tendrils into these clusters of diverse practice. Debbie Carson's naturopath, Kari, inspects Ethan's prescriptions. Van, a serious computer hobbyist since the 1980s, uses his computer to find health information, and has assembled a group of men to help him exercise and watch his weight. Rupal Patel consults his brother, a physician, to interpret biomedical data for him. Since the region contains a concentration of Indian immigrants, he can easily find a local Hindu temple to enhance his spiritual well-being. Clare was herself a *shiatsu* practitioner, and her company provides the ergonomic equipment she needs to be productive in light of her severe carpal tunnel syndrome.

Worker-centered Wellness Care

Worker-centered wellness care, the second great experiment, assumes that the individual workers are the locus of responsibility. In a joint research project, the Center for Disease Control and the Institute for the Future ascertained the relative determinants of health status: only 10 percent of illness can be accounted for by *access* to health care; 20 percent is based on genetics; another 20 percent stems from environmental factors; and a full half of a person's health status is explained by the behavior of individuals themselves (Johanson 2007, 43). Employers too are caught in this web because they have been the main avenue for health access to individual workers. Yet health-related costs are high and divert funds from other areas of capitalization. As noted in a Silicon Valley human resources conference featuring Cypress Semiconductors and Cisco, "[T]he root causes are obvious. Many of today's employees have a sense of passive entitlement to their benefits, are shielded from the real cost of the health care they consume, and [do not make] healthy lifestyle decisions based on their current risks and conditions" (Buck Consultants 2006). Given the current systemic constraints, employers cannot leverage changes in either the insurers to improve access or in making wholesale environmental changes, at least while keeping their costs low. Employers on the cutting edge shift their own policies from health *care* to health *promotion*, from disease management to behavioral change (Hymel 2006a).

Risk in contemporary society involves two intertwining concepts. It necessarily points to security and safety, but also to responsibility. The risks that stem, not from nature, but from our own modern life, carry responsibilities that point to layers of liability and ethical accountability (Giddens 1999, 7–9). However, those ethical duties are ambiguously distributed, falling to the state, employers, individuals, and their families. Living with the risk of chronic disease, that ultimate artifact of modernity, brings diverse ethical burdens to organizations and individuals. To the degree that stress and sedentary living are implied, workplaces are seen both as culpable and as sites for health improvement. Other behaviors are viewed as private, subject to individual, or at least familial, responsibility. The consequences, however, of those behaviors—translated into chronic disease burden—are felt in the workplace, especially as lost productivity and increased benefit costs. The complicated fiscal bond between employer and worker is at the heart of this dilemma.

The fracturing of risk-based third-party payment systems—that is, work-based health insurance—undermines health entitlements. Health care is increasingly expensive to employers, so they want to contain costs by limiting access. Additionally, workers change jobs, and companies come and go, making the ethical obligations of individual stakeholders that much more confusing. Even the definition of what constitutes a worker has changed. Is a contract worker employed through an agency entitled to benefits? The employer does not often do so. Agencies may offer benefit options, but rarely affordable ones.

In light of this ambiguity, organizations are experimenting with individuating work-based health care. Workers are "personally empowered" as the burden of care shifts to individuals to control their own behavior, and hence overall medical costs (Hogle 2005, 712). Chronic disease is closely linked with particular behaviors—smoking, being sedentary, overeating, and feeling negative emotions. Employers now focus on worker wellness to reward those workers who move, quit smoking, and substitute salads for steak. Companies give out pedometers to encourage workers to walk more. They provide stress reduction workshops and encourage an ethic of embodied emotional restraint and anger management. Here the condition of work is not the issue, but the condition of the *worker*. In a study of Canadian high-technology managers, sociologists MacEachen, Polzer, and Clarke (2008, 1026–27) note that managers promoted worker health to maintain productivity "even under intense and pressured conditions." Instead of worrying about organizational conditions, managers encouraged workers to build "resilience" so that they would be "able to withstand working conditions."

Health is political, with implications for the larger environment and civil order. As workers are "empowered" to control their own health, they will expect not only various alternative health options but also increasingly green ones. Catering to the health "empowerment" of individual workers is challenging. If managers spend time directing workers' efforts away from actual production, but instead take on the role of health coach, they are going beyond their competency. If companies spend time creating tools for health management and chronic disease prevention, they may trigger worker cynicism. The entire approach of worker wellness, however, assumes a sustainable relationship between company and worker and does not acknowledge the ephemerality of ties. Workers come and go—and temporary workers rarely even come into the equation. Seen from the other side, employers come and go and many can not be counted upon for care. Workers will find a way to create their own safety nets, if they can, but what was once seen as a given is now a source of resentment.

Moreover, the fundamental problem of inequality does not disappear with individually based strategies; rather it is intensified. Organizations are left with few options given the current realities of how risk is reckoned and distributed in the United States. Employers must drive workers to be healthier or abandon the work-based third-party payment system invented in the Great Depression. Building an infrastructure that gives access to wellness tools, not just late-in-illness access to emergency rooms, remains an issue. However, the intense productivity of the new economy depends not only on well workers but also on workers who can perform *better than well*. The new inequality will be built on the divisions between those who are allowed to participate in the knowledge economy as augmented producers, and those excluded from that world of wellness.

Elite workers already have ergonomic work situations, on-site gyms, and benefits designed to help them stay well, or *better than well*. Contract workers and other support personnel have yet to establish that their embodiment *counts*. They have not persuaded their contractors that such benefits could substantially improve their productivity. The instability of the employer-worker relationship, because of temporary employment status, short tenures, or company churn rates, makes it difficult to establish their embodiment as a reality. Organization must come to grips with the reality that working "brains-in-a-vat" have bodies.

In Silicon Valley, employers are trying employee-centered wellness programs that organizations hope will replace the increasingly expensive employee-based insurance system. In the last half-century, employers have been an engine for paying insurance premiums to repair the ills of physical and mental workers. As postinjury or disease intervention proves to be increasingly expensive, companies look to the less costly preventative care that will lead to worker sustainability. Worker-wellness programs maintain that keeping workers well is preferable (and potentially less expensive) than trying to fix ill, especially chronically ill, employees. Incentives are put in place to entice workers into this experiment. Bonuses are given to workers who take health assessments. Coaches are put in place to help workers change behaviors, such as smoking or being sedentary. Families are enlisted to become part of the change.

Organizations are attempting to become sites to encourage networked change as individual workers experiment with diverse practices and form communities of common healthy practice. Changes are tracked. Is weight lost? Are pedometers recording increased walking? Positive change is rewarded. For this system to work, employers must have a wider purview over the health of their embodied workers. There are also significant implications for organizations pursuing this strategy as the gaze of the organization goes beyond the workplace to a more holistic view of worker life. As households become sites of wellness and subject to tracking, criticism, and intervention by employers, work-home barriers will become even more thoroughly eroded.

Such pervasive reach evokes the **Panopticon**, an eighteenth-century prison design in which prisoners could always be observed. Michel Foucault used this metaphor to suggest the way the "scientifico-legal complex" from which power is derived observes and disciplines behavior (1995). The social bond between worker and employer may permit this gaze, but again, such a relationship is likely to be temporary. Contractors, subcontractors, temporary workers fall outside this "gaze," but are swept into it by virtue of their relationship to "real" workers. Both types of employee are gathered around the water cooler. If the permanent employee is being encouraged to eat vegetables while the contract worker at the next desk nibbles on donuts, the company's wellness work is for naught. Short tenure employment and the cynicism directed toward such "employee-centered" efforts undermine the sustainability of healthful practices.

The social world of families is recognized, albeit partially, by organizational human resources personnel who grapple with the dilemma of work-home "balance." The continued erosion of the barriers around the modules of work, home, and health extend the power of the workplace even more deeply into family life. Worker wellness can be effective only in well families. Concomitantly, the family members are more deeply involved with workplaces as diet, embodied movement and posture patterns, attitudes about self, and optimism shape the productivity of the worker. Homes, workplaces, and health care sites are becoming less fixed. People live, work, and do personal health care in multiple sites from automobiles to gardens. Modules of work, home, and health are being recast and reshuffled so that tightly compartmentalized living is becoming increasingly difficult. Those born to this environment favor it, while their elders struggle with lost metaphors and a sense that they are being hounded by their mobile phones. For organizations, work-home initiatives and wellness enterprises must be connected; putting these efforts into separate initiatives would render them less effective. Effective efforts, however, would mean a substantial rethinking of the social contract between employee and employer. Privacy is an artifact of a different social agreement.

If organizations are successful in reorganizing health benefits of employee-centered wellness initiatives, this will compound the problems experienced by marginal, new, and retired workers in the current insurance system. Risk will be increasingly differentiated, with one category of worker, the directly employed long-term worker, benefiting from improved health, while those at the margin without these wellness programs grow more risky to insure. It is conceivable that networks will take new tasks on themselves, forming platforms for health benefits. We already have existing examples of actors with unstable work forming a professional guild to shift risk and get health benefits. Guilds, unions, professional associations, staffing firms, and alumni associations could well experiment with these new wellness-centered benefit plans in ways that would minimize the responsibilities of individual employers (Malone 2004, 84–89). Although unionization is more problematic, Silicon Valley workers have already demonstrated their ability to form professional, ethnic, and professional-ethnic network associations, making that scenario quite plausible.

Moreover, the new discourses of work morality, especially ones of **corporate social responsibility** (CSR), require that the abstracted workers-in-a-vat must be put back into their bodies and into their worlds. CSR tenets demand that organizations acknowledge a triple bottom line beyond mere money, including impacts on people and the planet. That position is an inherently embodied philosophy. In the past, customers were also entities for whom corporate responsibility for their welfare was limited; they were once as "disembodied" in the organizational mind as numbers. The emerging philosophy of corporate social responsibility suggests that customers too must be recognized as valid social entities. While corporate social responsibility can easily become a cynical exercise in brand image improvement, it is also a major reconceptualization of the social contract of capitalism.

In the philosophy of corporate social responsibility, shareholders are not the only people who matter—workers and customers, and the communities in which they reside, must be reckoned in the accounting. The literal physical environment in which they move must also be considered. The minimal social contract strives to make worker conditions and communities less toxic—driving a new industry in green design and building. The greening of products and services recognizes that customers too live in bodies in the world. This philosophy may create new opportunities for entrepreneurs. As the first decade of the twenty-first century unfolds, Silicon Valley is poised again at a conscious reinvention of itself to become the innovator and purveyor of green technology. That greening of technology will feed back into notions of health and health care, adding to the pool of diverse medical beliefs.

Deep Medical Diversity

The third experiment taking place in Silicon Valley is deep medical diversity. Fundamental to deep diversity is the concept of deep toleration, being "open to the possibility that [their] values might not be the best ones available to them at a given point and time." People practicing deep toleration consider "that the contrasting moral sources of others might offer a better language of self-interpretation than the moral sources one presently relies upon" (Redhead 2002b, 816). In other words, it is possible to learn not only different practices from other cultures but also even moral frameworks for self-actualization. The intensity and density of cultural differences, born of ancestral and experimental identities, drives people either into deep toleration or to the isolation of intolerance. Silicon Valley people—at least the culturally effective ones— cannot rush to judgment, but must consider and adjust to the fact that there really are significantly different ways to be in the world. In the context of health, such toleration supports the search for practices and narratives that better reflect the embodied worker who is escaping the fetters of Descartes' duality of body and mind. Companies might well seriously consider mining their employees' diverse wellness practices for those that can be more widely used by other employees. To do this they would need to develop criteria to assess the effectiveness of the practices based on the epistemology of productive embodiment, not necessarily the statistical metrics of normality and disease.

In the absence of institutional support, there is already a lively informal economy of trading traditional and alternative medical practices. Out-of-pocket expenses may be converted to service exchanges. Massages can be traded for organic garden produce. Chinese medicinal herbs are brought as gifts from visiting relatives. Online support groups facilitate transactions as individuals collect, evaluate, and disseminate experiences. Some websites become central distribution nodes, just as Mendosa.com, *Living with Diabetes*, became a clearinghouse for the diabetic community. David Mendosa took his own experience with the disease and reshaped his career as a science writer to inspect and disseminate information to anyone who needs it.

Within health care plans workers take the initiative to work around institutional restrictions to seek out alternative care. If the wife's medical plan allows for acupuncture and the husband's does not, the couple makes sure that her plan, not his, is used to experiment with pain alleviation. As the practices of deep medical diversity proliferate, workers will continue to pressure organizations to support their experiments. Organizations would be wise to ready themselves for these changes.

Deep diversity, in the guise of deep medical diversity, poses opportunities and challenges for organizations. Health maintenance organizations, insurance companies, and other employer-pay organizations are currently oriented around biomedicine. They are the pinnacle of statistical epistemology; clinical trials are the gold standard for acceptable and payable practices. The diagnostic discovery of biomedical disease etiology must be followed by the accepted therapy in a way that maximizes the statistical probability of success and minimizes risks. American health care, especially that funded by health insurance, is built upon these assumptions. However, wellness is more epistemologically agnostic. If a practice works, people will use it. Yoga, *taiji*, ChiRunning, and hiking with the Sierra Club are all active; these practices require movement, whatever their sociocultural origins. Politicized vegan or Brahmin vegetarian diets avoid the dreaded American red meat diet and are in alignment with the American Heart Association. The scope of wellness is much broader than that of illness, which requires therapeutic intervention to "fix" problems. If employers are going to foster employee-centered wellness programs, they must seriously contemplate harnessing the deep medical diversity that their employees already practice. Some Silicon Valley organizations hint at this already. Remember Jeremy Fitzgerald's work-site yoga class and Margot's work as a massage therapist at the high-tech campus? But what of practices that have not yet swept into everyday acceptance?: Chinese medicinal meals, Vietnamese spirit mediums, herbs from Latino *botánicas*. Workers use these practices on themselves, but without the knowledge or acknowledgement of employers. As workplaces move to an emphasis on wellness, they will encounter more deep medical diversity; but they lack the tools to evaluate their effectiveness.

There is a clear analogy for this in the environmental movement and how it has reckoned with risks. In Europe in the 1980s, in order to prevent policy paralysis, a **precautionary principle** was adopted. This rule suggested that "action on environmental issues (and by inference other forms of risk) should be taken even though there is scientific uncertainty about them"

(Giddens 1999, 9). Wellness initiatives, by sweeping in individuals with their broad repertoire of practices, find themselves inadvertently adopting a <u>precautionary principle</u> of their own in order to change behavior broadly connected to health. Engineers get massages from Margot, through direct contract with the company's health provider. However, by granting individuals the burden of care, they are also indirectly supporting Celia as she works on deficient kidney meridians or contemplates a client's connection to the Daoist spirit world.

Naturalistic medical traditions, upon which both immigrant and alternative practices are based, were once called "empirical medical traditions." If a practice worked on a person, that story became part of the greater body of lore. Knowledge was not validated by statistics, but stories. This herb worked, that massage did not. Scientists would scathingly remark that this approach uses anecdotal evidence; insurance providers reject the approach. However, this is exactly the sort of narrative people use in their networks to validate a particular practice. If organizations learn practices of deep medical diversity from their workers, they will need to organize and vet these stories, much as David Mendosa finds practices for managing diabetes and filters them through the lens of endocrinology to eliminate practices that would do harm.

Trajectories

In the nineteenth century a pattern was already forming in the San Francisco Bay Area. As a gateway for immigrants, the region grew diverse in cuisine, language, and commercial experimentation. The area was a magnet for utopian seekers toying with self-conscious reinventions ranging from classic Emersonian Transcendentalism to socialism. Even the institutions that were created in the region—the Bank of Italy (later the Bank of America), Stanford, and the University of California—deviated from accepted practice. Among the many social experiments was a merger of two diverse values—a reverence for nature and a utopian vision of technological efficiency. The underlying optimism of this *ethos* fueled continued social tinkering. It is not surprising that the health culture that emerged over a century later would reflect the complexity of immigrant cultures and the deliberate utopianism of alternative experimentation.

Silicon Valley, in this regard, is very much a part of the larger health culture, but with a unique twist. That piece of transcendental experimentation given to technological optimism grew disproportionately in the South Bay. Along with federal investment in research and development infrastructure, scientists and technologists were searching for a larger purpose to which this knowledge would be put.

The countercultural experiments that began in the 1950s pushed the direction of technological innovation toward augmentation, a master metaphor that would change the direction of computing. Self-actualization, augmentation, and self-management were master practices that would integrate the larger Bay Area health culture into the emerging work culture of Silicon Valley. Embodiment for productivity would become a dominant *habitus*, as would an *ethos* of continual self-experimentation.

The Fourth Wave

Silicon Valley's health culture has been defined by particular themes:

- The health *ethos* reflects the distinctive work culture of the *place*.
- *Experimentation* is embraced in many arenas of life, including bodily practices.
- People work, live, and seek health in a *deeply medically diverse* environment that combines sophisticated biomedical approaches with countercultural and immigrant-based modalities.
- The *restaging* of work, family, and health means that each age cohort experiences the health culture a bit differently.
- Individuals, families, and whole communities experience an increased *burden of empowerment*—as they bear the brunt of the productivity ethic, sacrificing or augmenting health in order to keep functioning.

The changes that have occurred over the past decades to hone this *ethos* have implications for the future.

Silicon Valley's significance as a place is not etched in stone. Yet peo-

ple are drawn to it, or born into it, and thereby enact a particular identity—entrepreneurial, technologically optimistic, and creative. Whether the
region becomes the heart of innovative green technology is yet to be determined, yet the struggle to *reinvent* itself is part of the distinctive quality of
the region. The iconic value of the region is reinforced by repeated stories
of triumph that, although hyperbole, have the power to influence people
locally and globally. If it reinvents itself again, future waves of people will
fashion a worldview that builds on American transcendental values—augmentation, respect for nature, and optimism regarding human potential.
These values continue to inform the health culture of the region—more so
with each passing generational wave.

Experimentation will continue as people use their bodies as media for
artistic expression of their social identities. The bodies of the first and even
second wave are aging, and they make sincere efforts to age well, or at least
less visibly. The third wave cohort, who are still young, use their bodies to
signal their ever-changing identities. Cosmetic neurology, body modification, and medically diverse experimentation are comfortable media for them.
New medical technologies, global fashions, and Internet-based access to a
global marketplace will intensify this experimentation in the **fourth wave**.

The countercultural encounters with other people's medical traditions
have been reinforced by the presence of immigrant-based practices. The
second, and particularly the youngest third wave, have grown to accept that
a diversity of health images, agents, and practices is available and can be
used experimentally. The fluid integration of countercultural yoga with
immigrant Indo-American cultural practices "Indianizes" the health marketplace. Similarly, the presence of Chinese grandmothers publicly practicing *taiji* or picking up ginkgo fruits at dawn "Sinocizes" the corpus of
available alternative activities for Chinese and non-Chinese alike. The deep
medical diversity of that complex health market reflects the larger deep
diversity of the Californian urban landscape, and will only escalate. Premises and practices will become progressively intermixed. A new version of
"wellness" will emerge in the fourth wave, informed by cross-cultural interactions, transcendental notions, and pragmatic cost-saving organizational
practices.

The restaging of work-life phases is already underway. The first wave was socialized to believe that education took place in youth, to be replaced by paid work and finally rewarded with a recreationally filled retirement. While that vision did not quite materialize for them, as it had appeared to do for the Silent Generation, it was still an ideal. The second wave watched that ideal evaporate, and the youngest third wave scoffs at the sequence, snorting skeptically if they hear the phrase "Social Security" used in reference to their own futures. In the new economy, education, skill, experience, and security are not to be taken for granted. Instead, people are expected to make themselves flexible, adaptable, and capable of weathering market forces. This individuation of productivity intruded into the expectations of the oldest first wave but is becoming increasingly natural to the cohorts that followed them. The fourth wave will take it for granted.

So what can we anticipate for the fourth wave, the children and grandchildren of the previous generations? How will Kristal's and Jeremy's children view themselves within their ecosystem of complex cultures, shifting work patterns, and expectations for healthy productivity? What will Ethan's imagined offspring value? They will have been born in a time of global economic and climatic redefinition. Yet, we can expect that some of the changes that have occurred from the first to the third wave will continue. The fourth wave, the next cohort to come, will grow up in a cultural environment in which the body-mind-spirit is a fluid continuum, not such distinctly professionally segregated silos—the mind the province of psychologists, the body given to physicians to attend. This wave will exert effort to craft themselves into interesting, productive beings, but ones that will differ even from those we now identify as digital natives. They will be drawing on diverse cultural practices that will become more and more divorced from ancestral cultures. In other words, one does not have to be born of Chinese or Latino parents to cheerfully lift practices and elements of identity from those cultural categories. Ethnogenesis, the creation of new culture, through mash-ups of existing and imaginary cultures, will seem increasingly natural to the fourth wave. Health policy pundits, human resources specialists, and science journalists will link behavior to health even more tightly. Consequently, behavior modification will be seen as the critical path to health. Pressure for such modification will come from families, friends, workplaces, media, and politics. Tinkering with the behavioral self will become fashion, augmented by a host of social technologies. The fundamental relationship of government, employer, and health will change for them. The behavior modification to which they will subject themselves will be less regulated by professional and governmental licensing, but still subject to other controlling processes such as technological monitoring, fashion, and lifelong education.

Individuals in the fourth cohort will describe themselves by mixing an ethereal vocabulary of "wellness" with a halo of medical metrics, the result of less expensive and more readily available monitoring devices. This mixture of health metaphors and metrics will be shared through consumer-generated media and will become a critical element of one's identity. Faith in technology will not disappear, but will become individualized and perhaps less visible as it penetrates and adorns the body, extends the mind, and rationalizes the spirit. The coupling of health and productivity, which began with Silicon Valley's first wave of revolutionaries, will even more profoundly define the fourth wave. Silicon Valley, reflecting both core American values and global trends, might once again be a bellwether for a recasting of what constitutes "being and well-being."

Glossary

Glossary

AARP: Formerly the American Association of Retired People, a nonprofit service provider and lobbyist for people over fifty

ADHD; attention deficit hyperactivity disorder: The most commonly diagnosed childhood psychiatric disorder in which problems with attention are linked with hyperactivity

affirmations: Repeated statements that reinforce positive thinking

aging well: Aging with a minimum of health problems and a strong sense of well-being

American Transcendentalism: A group of ideas that emerged in New England in the nineteenth century that valued nature, romantic spiritualism, an experimental approach to life, and draws on romantic versions of Asian thought or Orientalism

animism: A belief that natural entities have consciousness or spirits that are subject to human intervention

animatism: A belief in a generalized impersonal power over which people have some control

anime: An abbreviation for fictional hand-drawn and computer animation from Japan

augmentation; augmented: Using technology, foods, pharmaceuticals, body modifications, and other cultural practices to enhance oneself and increase productivity

Ayurvedic; Ayurvedic medicine: The nearly three-thousand-year-old system of medical beliefs and practices from the Indian subcontinent that are used globally as a form of alternative medicine

Beats: A groups of writers who came to prominence in the 1950s, often associated with the San Francisco Renaissance, and who later evolved into the 1960s counterculture

better than well: The state of seeking health beyond the simple absence of illness

biomedicine; biomedical: The theory and knowledge of medicine connected to the biosciences and chemistry that is the basis of the practice of rationalistic, scientific medicine

body modifications: A range of cross-cultural practices including tattooing, piercing, and surgical augmentation for artistic and cultural reasons

***botánicas*:** A retail store that sells folk and alternative medicine, largely within the Latino/Latina community

breast pump: A device used to pump human breast milk for storage and later use

carpal tunnel: A passageway of bony and fibrous tissue on the palm side of the wrist, and a shortened phrase referring to carpal tunnel syndrome, a painful chronic condition in which the median nerve is compressed

Cartesian dualism: The notion, associated with seventeenth-century French philosopher René Descartes, that the observing mind is separate from the machinelike body

chiropractic; chiropractor: A medical system in which malaise stems from the misalignment of the bones, especially the vertebra, which can then be manipulated into the proper position

ChiRunning: An exercise form that applies the principles of *taiji*, such as meditative awareness, balance, and controlled breathing, to running

ChiWalking: An exercise form that applies the principles of *taiji*, such as meditative awareness, balance, and controlled breathing, to walking

chronic disease burden: The impact of long-term behaviorally based diseases in terms of cost, mortality, and morbidity

churn rate: High employee turnover or a high rate of business failure and creation

clean room: A room kept free of airborne particles, including dust, skin flakes, microbes, and chemical vapors, in order to manufacture sensitive precision components

coaches; life coaching: Educating and guiding individuals to change their lives based on future goals

cognitive diversity: Having different ways and styles of thinking

cohort: Sometimes referred to popularly as "generations," a group of people of similar age who have had distinct common experiences

complementary and alternative medicine; CAM: Practices that integrate folk, naturalistic, and New Age healing practices with biomedicine or provide alternatives to them

contingent workers: Independent professional, consultant, and temporary contract workers who are not direct employees of the organization with which they work

contract worker; contractors: A subset of the contingent workforce that is contracted to work on a specific project

coronary artery disease; CAD: The end result of a blockage of the coronary arteries that supply the myocardium heart muscle

corporate social responsibility; CSR: A business philosophy in which private organizations accept responsibility for the impact of their activities on employees, consumers, the natural environment, and the public at large

cosmetic neurology: Using pharmaceuticals to move individuals from one normal cognitive state to another preferred one

cosmetic surgery: Altering a normal body to a preferred state through surgery

countercultural: A sociological term that describes a group that seeks a sociocultural existence different than the mainstream

cultural competencies: Refers to the ability to move successfully between cultures and understand and act within their differences

curanderos: Folk healers within Latino communities who use practices that draw on a wide variety of indigenous shamanistic traditions and European naturalistic beliefs

deep diversity: A term coined to refer to significant, complex, and nonobvious cultural differences that characterize people of a particular political unit or region

deep medical diversity: The state of significant, complex, and nonobvious pluralism in which people draw on different medical beliefs and practices, some from immigrant ancestral traditions and others from hybrid biomedical and alternative ones

diabetes: A disease state in which people do not produce enough insulin, or do not properly respond to it, in order to metabolize glucose into energy

dialysis: A medical procedure employing a device to replace the water and waste removal functions of the kidney, using diffusion across a semipermeable membrane

digital natives: Refers to those born after the widespread use of digital technologies to whom the practices and uses of devices are integrated into everyday life

disruptive technology: Providing products or services that the market does not expect and that provide new arenas of development

Elephant Pharmacy: An integrated alternative and medical pharmacy that served the San Francisco Bay Area between 2003 and 2009. It was similar to Pharmaca Integrative Pharmacy stores based out of Boulder, Colorado

embodied: Knowledge that resides in the body in a social and cultural milieu

embrained: Knowledge presumed to exist in the brain

emotion work: Disciplining body, mind, and behavior to school emotions to match the expectations of the social setting

employee-centered wellness programs: Public and private efforts designed to improve the behaviors known to be associated with chronic disease in order to prevent expensive interventions

encoded knowledge: Knowledge that is written down

enhancement medicine: Medicine that is less focused on cure than enhancing normal experiences

epistemology; medical epistemology: The forms of knowledge relating to medical thought including assumptions, foundational beliefs, and reasoning processes

est; Erhard Seminars Training: Self-help programs developed by Werner Erhard that were popular between 1971 and 1984, which used trainers to facilitate self-revelation

ethnogenesis: The creation of new cultural practices and schema

ethnomathematics: The cultural beliefs and practices about numeracy and numerical logic that differ from culture to culture

ethnoscapes: A term coined by Arjun Appadurai to refer to the transnational movement of peoples

ethos: The attitudes, practices, and habits of a group, time period, or cultural context, from the Greek for "custom" and "disposition"

etiology: The causes of disease

feng shui: A form of geomancy drawing on Chinese Daoist principles to improve one's life through the articulation of the built environment with the natural world

first wave; first wave cohort: Members of the cohort born in the decades after World War II, 1946 to 1964, colloquially referred to as Baby Boomers

formulary: In pharmaceutical practices, a listing of prescriptions approved for use

fourth wave; fourth wave cohort: The age cohort born in the twenty-first century, who are children of the second and third wave age cohorts

functional foods: Foods designed, or claiming, to have disease-reducing and health-promoting properties

Gaia: A philosophy that life on the earth is a single coevolving system, perhaps imbued with consciousness, and an anime-themed social gaming site

Ganesha: A Hindu, Buddhist, and Jain deity with the head of an elephant, who is revered as the "Remover of Obstacles"

Gestalt therapy: A process developed by Dick Price and Fritz and Laura Perls at Esalen Institute to promote an awareness of the unity of behavior, affect, and self

GLBTQ: Gay, Lesbian, Bisexual, Transsexual, and Queer, referring to a variety of sexual orientations that contrast to heterosexuality

glucometer: A glucose meter, a device for measuring the amount of glucose in the blood

governmentality: A concept first developed by the French social theorist Michel Foucault and refined by Nikolas Rose that refers to the organized practices, including ways of thinking and techniques, through which people are governed and disciplined

habitus: A concept developed by Marcel Mauss and refined by Pierre Bourdieu, referring to the structures of mind related to a set of tastes, dispositions, and beliefs particular to a grouping of people

health cultures: The aspects of belief, practice, and *habitus* related to health in particular groups of people

health ethic: A form of work ethic in which mental, physical, and spiritual disciplines are applied to the crafting of self to improve well-being

health span: An emerging public health concept referring to the number of years you can live relatively free of serious disease

health maintenance organization; HMO: A type of managed medical care organization that provides health care coverage to members in the United States, often to large organizational clients, such as Kaiser Permanente or CIGNA Health Care

holistic health: A hybrid set of practices based on merging popular psychology with naturalistic medical traditions from Native America, Europe, and East and South Asia

Homebrew Computer Club: A hobbyist computer group that began to meet in Menlo Park in the 1970s and included the founders of many microcomputer companies, including Apple

homeopathy; homeopathic: A form of alternative medicine associated with the eighteenth-century German physician Samuel Hahnemann that prepares and administers unique diluted preparations that are thought to cause effects similar to the symptoms presented

illness narrative: A form of ethnographic writing used to describe the experiences of people as they live through health and illness to illustrate larger cultural issues in medical anthropology

immanent: A metaphysical concept in which the spiritual infuses into what would otherwise be considered mundane

intensification: A concept in political and economic anthropology to describe the heightened effort required to keep production at a high level

kanpo: Chinese medicine as practiced in Japan

kidney meridian: In Chinese medicine, this channel for *qi* energy is the "Minister for Power," a reservoir for energy related to the kidney system that includes the adrenals; it runs from the little toe to the root of the tongue

life staging: The cultural division of life into childhood, adolescence, young and middle adulthood, and old age with associated expectations for appropriate behavior

manga: A Japanese or Japanese-style graphic novel

Marfan's syndrome: A hereditary disorder that affects the connective tissues with implications for limb length and heart health

materia medica: The term used to refer to the knowledge and practices around any substance used for healing

McJobs: Low-paying jobs that offer little chance of advancement and require few skills

medical epistemologies: The forms of knowledge relating to medical thought including assumptions, foundational beliefs, and reasoning processes

medical pluralism: The term most commonly used in medical anthropology to refer to the use of more than one medical system, including biomedicine, traditional, and alternative hybrid systems for healing

Medicare Part D: A federal program for subsidizing prescription drug costs for patients in the Medicare system

meridians: In traditional Chinese medicine (TCM), these are the channels for the flow of *qi* energy that can be influenced by acupressure, acupuncture, *qigong*, or moxabustion

Merry Pranksters: A group of people associated with Ken Kesey in the 1960s that combined communal living, psychedelic experimentation, and technological optimism, including Steward Brand

modularity: In cognitive anthropology, this concept refers to the tendency to break complex thoughts, behaviors, and built systems into discrete components

multiple chemical sensitivity; MCS: This syndrome refers a persistent set of symptoms induced by exposure to low levels of chemicals

narcolepsy: A sleep disorder characterized by excessive daytime sleepiness

natural food: An elastic and symbolic category for food that has undergone minimal processing

Naturalistic etiologies: Causes of disease, including environmental, humoral, and emotional imbalance, common to the naturalistic medical systems that developed in ancient East Asia, South Asia, and Europe

naturopathy; naturopathic: An alternative medical system that focuses on natural remedies and assumes the body's ability to heal itself with minimal surgical or pharmaceutical intervention

Neopets: A virtual pets website for subscribers

neurolinguistic programming; NLP: A controversial therapeutic approach for self and organizational change linking successful behavior to underlying patterns of thought

nutraceuticals: This category includes supplements and functional foods, nutritional products that aspire to health benefits beyond their quantified nutritional value

neuropathy: This term refers to diseases of the nerves or side effects from systemic diseases, primarily affecting the legs and feet

New Age: A decentralized social movement that includes a hybrid set of practices and beliefs designed to maximize human potential

new economy: A term that encompasses the economic changes of globalization and a shift to a service-sector, asset-based economy, particularly associated with pervasive high technology and information exchange

otaku: a dedicated fan of anime, manga, and video gaming, a neutral descriptor outside of Japan but derogatory inside

Panopticon: An architectural style of prison design in which prisoners can be watched without knowing whether they are being observed. Michel Foucault expanded its meaning metaphorically

personal health ecology, personal health ecologies: A phrase used by the Institute for the Future to describe the flow of health beliefs and practices in and through a person's social network

pragmatism: A philosophical view that a concept should be evaluated on how well it works and a metaphor for valuing practicality

precautionary principle: A policy concept that suggests that scientific uncertainty should not forestall action that may protect the environment

psoriasis: A chronic noncontagious inflammation of the skin or joints, possibly autoimmune in origin

qigong: A practice of breath, movement, and meditation associated with Daoist practices and traditional Chinese medicine

qualitative; qualitative metrics of health: Assessing health through subjective criteria such as perceptions of vitality, mood, and pain

quantitative; quantitative metrics of health: Assessing health status by measuring objective criteria such as blood glucose, blood pressure, or body weight

risk pools; risk pooling: Refers to the grouping of people insured; large pools can spread the risk and small pools can be manipulated to include the most healthy and least risky population

second wave; second wave cohort: People born after the first wave cohort, roughly from 1961 to 1981, although precise dates of birth differ for those colloquially called "Generation X"

self-actualization: Although it has specific meanings in psychology, it also refers to a general humanistic approach that promotes health and motivates people to determine and act on their individual potential

sexual liberation: A term popularized in the 1960s and 1970s to refer to a social shift toward open discussions of the political context of sexual repression

shivambu kalpa: The therapeutic use of urine, through topical application and oral consumption, in Indian Ayurvedic medical practices

sleep apnea: A sleep disorder in which the person pauses breathing while asleep

social imaginary: The historical or cultural constructs that provide meaning for a particular social grouping

somaticization: Internalizing emotions or other sensations in the body

Straight Edge; sXers; Straight Edgers: A youth-based social movement associated with hardcore punk rock music in which alcohol, tobacco, recreational drugs, and casual sexual encounters are to be avoided, sometimes associated with vegan diet and animal rights activism; it is marked with the symbol "X"

street racing; street race: Unsanctioned car racing on public roads, although some communities sponsor events to provide an alternative to illegal racing

structural violence: Systematic ways in which social structures and institutions (sexism, racism, and so forth) reduce life chances

superfund site: A place in which hazardous waste is abandoned and no responsible party can be found, so that the federal government is directed to use special funds to clean the site. The official name is the Comprehensive Environmental Response, Compensation, and Liability Act of 1980

sustainability: An economic and political philosophy in which environments, practices, and products have the capacity to endure

taijiquan; taiji: A martial art from China that has been exported as a meditative exercise regime

temporary workers: Employees contracted for work on a temporary basis and not given the same rights and privileges as permanent employees

third wave; third wave cohort: An age group born between the mid-1980s and the 1990s with various popular names such as Generation Y, the Millennial Generation, and the Echo Boom, the youngest of whom are digital natives

traditional Chinese medicine; TCM: The set of principles and practices related to healing, with origins in China, including acupuncture, dietary therapy, acupressure massage, and herbal treatments

vegan: A person who avoids animal products of any kind in clothing and diet, including eggs, dairy, and honey, which are sometimes used by less stringent vegetarians

web 2.0 companies: Organizations that promote a more democratic relationship between software developers and end-users who generate content for the application, including wikis, blogs, and social networking websites

Weight Watchers: An international company that provides dieting services and products to members, largely focused on tracking foods by fat, calories, and fiber

Whole Foods Market: A chain of grocery stores, based out of Texas, that retail "natural" products and a mix of organically and conventionally grown produce

Wii game consoles: A home game console by Nintendo that uses a wireless remote to detect motion and direct the action of the game

xiyi: The Chinese word, in Pinyin, for "Western" biomedicine

zhongyi: The Chinese word, in Pinyin, for traditional Chinese medicine

Notes

Preface and Acknowledgments

1. Throughout this book pseudonyms are used to protect the identities of people who participated in the project. Confidentiality is further protected by masking the person's employer. Only those people well established in the public sector are given their actual names.

Chapter 1: Embodying Place

EPIGRAPH: "11th Chorus" was originally published in *Book of Blues* by Jack Kerouac ©1995, Penguin Poets. Reprinted with the permission of SLL/Sterling Lord Literistic, Inc. Copyright by Jack Kerouac.

1. Linguistically, nearly half—48 percent—of the total population speaks a language other than English at home, and nearly half of those households, 49 percent, speak an Asian or Pacific Islander language (U.S. Census Bureau 2005; Henton et al. 2008, 10). In the United States as a whole, 20 percent speak a language other than English (U.S. Census Bureau 2006b). In the categories of the U.S. census, "race" and language underscore potential cultural differences in which people bring a rich range of medical beliefs and practices into the region. Interactions by multiple cultures imply new challenges for care delivery. Schools are not the only public sites where an English language infrastructure is challenged by linguistic diversity; every public clinic has the same situation.

Within the family, the faith traditions of one's ancestors may or may not endure. A bilingual national study of religion in the United States revealed that while only 7 percent of respondents were unaffiliated as children, by the time they emerge from their teens, 20 percent declare themselves unaffiliated (Lugo et al. 2008, 5, 23). This pool of people, who enter and exit institutionalized religion as consumers, is even larger in the western United States (ibid., 8). Santa Clara County itself offers many platforms for religious experience—including more than 200 churches for Protestants, 55 for Catholics, 55 for Latter-Day Saints, 17 Jewish temples and synagogues, 10 mosques, 32 Buddhist temples, 6 temples for Sikhs, 14 for Baha'i, and 15 for Hindus (Center for Religious and Civic Culture 2008). Religious organizations run 15 percent of the nonprofit organizations in Silicon Valley (Rafter and Silverman 2006, 44). These institutions work in subtle ways in Silicon Valley's immigrant-heavy demography. For example, in her study of a Californian Taiwanese immigrant church, sociologist Carolyn Chen notes that it is difficult to maintain the Confucian family–centered household in America. Taiwanese families convert to Christianity and place Christ in the center of the family, experiencing a religious piety that preserves the traditional centrality of family but allows parents to adopt a friendlier, less authoritarian role than that defined by Confucian filial piety (2002).

2. In popular culture, a cohort—a group of people of the same age that have a common experience—is often represented by the word "generation." Although the term is widely used in academic and popular discourse, I am uncomfortable with the fast and loose usage of the word "generation" to refer to age groupings, or cohorts. In the sixties, the "Boomer" cohort focused on the generation gap that seemed to divide them from their parents' generation, reifying the word "generation" (Roszak 2001, 137). After that epiphany, age groupings were all called "generation": "Silent Generation," "Generation X," "Generation Y," the "Millennial Generation." However, this conflation of age groups and generations can be confusing and misleading. Moreover, each of these terms has become stereotypic, loaded with self-congratulatory or denigrating discourse. These "generational" terms will be rarely used here, but instead will be represented as specific cohorts.

3. Margaret Lock, whose work ranges from Japanese conceptions of menopause to the cultural conceptions of death, summarizes the anthropological scholarship on embodiment in her 1993 *Annual Review of Anthropology* article "Cultivating the Body: Anthropology and Epistemologies of Bodily Practice and Knowledge." Later, she was one of the contributors in the themed edi-

tion of *Body and Society* (2001, volume 7, number 2)—along with such medical anthropologists as Lawrence Cohen and Nancy Scheper-Hughes—which explores how bodies are converted to capital. In 2007, Lock and Judith Farquhar published an edited volume, *Beyond the Body Proper*, dedicated to reincorporating the body in a social analysis.

Chapter 2: Wearable Parts

EPIGRAPH: "True Night" was originally published in *Axe Handles: Poems* by Gary Snyder ©1983, North Point Press. Reprinted with permission.

1. "Biocitizenship" is a concept that has emerged from the Foucauldian reassertion of health and health care into a larger political and economic context. Health issues are intrinsically political, and as citizens view such health-related issues as questions of power and inequality, they can be redefined as biocitizens. The notion of biocitizen implies active engagement with the politics of health care—the distribution of pharmaceuticals, the ecology of nutritional and environmental resources, and access to care.

2. While key figures—such as Dr. Zhen or Jerry Allen Johnson—are well-known public figures, other medical *qigong* practitioners who were observed and interviewed ethnographically have been given pseudonyms. The "Enduring Pine Healing Center" is based on an existing medical *qigong* center in San Jose, but one that goes by another name.

3. Michael Goldstein addresses the different approaches to mind and body inherent in alternative and biomedicine in the second chapter of his book *Alternative Health Care* (1999). Hans Baer's books, *Biomedicine and Alternative Healing Systems in America* and *Toward an Integrative Medicine: Merging Alternative Therapies with Biomedicine*, are two of the major works of critical medical anthropology on the subject of CAM, complementary and alternative medicine (2001a; 2004). His examination of the relationship between holistic and biomedical practices and institutions is particularly important for understanding deep medical diversity.

Chapter 3: In Production

EPIGRAPHS: *The Little Red Hen* by Florence White Williams was originally published in 1918. Excerpts included in this volume were taken from Project

Gutenberg, 2006. http://www.gutenberg.org/files/18735/18735.txt (accessed December 23, 2009). "Untitled Poem" was originally published in *Axe Handles: Poems* by Gary Snyder ©1983, North Point Press. Reprinted with permission.

Chapter 4: Gearing Up

EPIGRAPH: "46th Chorus" was originally published in *Book of Blues* by Jack Kerouac ©1995, Penguin Poets. Reprinted with the permission of SLL/Sterling Lord Literistic, Inc. Copyright by Jack Kerouac.

1. In the Institute for the Future project in which John Carter was interviewed and shadowed in Silicon Valley, cross-cultural interviews were conducted in London, Stockholm, Tokyo, and Helsinki. Straight Edge played a role for identity formation and embodied discipline both in Silicon Valley and in London (Gorbis et al. 2001).

2. Redbull is one of a suite of energy drinks aimed at the young. With 80 grams of caffeine, this drink, marketed as having mythical origins in Bangkok, "gives you wings" (Reid 2005, 8, 17).

Chapter 5: Structural Failure

EPIGRAPH: "Winter Almond" was originally published in *Danger on Peaks: Poems* by Gary Snyder ©2004, Shoemaker Hoard. Reprinted with permission.

1. While the per capita income is 57 percent higher than the national average, the cost of living is 47 percent higher. A two-worker household budget needs to be over U.S.$77,076 to meet basic needs in this region (Henton et al. 2008, 22). According to the 2006 Census Bureau breakdowns, more than 40 percent of the households live under that number, compared with the 6.5 percent that live under the official poverty line. The average monthly mortgage is $2,798, compared with the U.S. average of $1,402—although that number is volatile given the unstable housing market (U.S. Census Bureau 2006a; U.S. Census Bureau 2006b). While theaverage rent in the United States is only $763, in Santa Clara County apartment rents peaked in 2008 at $1,708 a month, and then dropped to $1,536 in 2009 (McAllister and Carey 2009).

2. Some 26 percent of Santa Clara County's middle and high school students are overweight or at risk of being overweight (Fenstersheib 2007). Depression rates for adolescents are reflected in the following 2007 statistics: 24 percent

of deaths among Latino and African American youth are due to homicide, 15 percent of teen deaths are due to suicide, and a full 19 percent of young people contemplated seriously hurting themselves (ibid., 42; Reyes and Cheng 2001, 89).

3. In Santa Clara County, nearly half, 48 percent, of people over sixty-five do not have enough income to meet their most basic needs. Fifty-five percent of the older women, 81 percent of older Latinos, and 77 per cent of Asian elders struggle economically. Unlike the rest of California, owning a house in Silicon Valley may only add to the burden of the elderly, not relieve it (Insight Center for Community Economic Development 2009). While 70 percent of health care insurance for people under sixty-five is still obtained through the workplace, that number is dropping as private insurance becomes a more direct household purchase (Henton et al. 2007, 30–31). Private insurance is the option for those nontraditionally employed people who can afford any insurance. The 2007 overall rate of public and private medical coverage is 84 percent in the United States, and 87 percent in Santa Clara County. Gay Becker (2004, 258–59) reports that on a national level, teenagers, unemployed workers, persons fifty-five to sixty-four, and ethnic minorities dominate the numbers of the uninsured. Wage earners without health benefits are also at risk for incurring illness without coverage. Continuous coverage would mean a national decrease in mortality of from 5 to 15 percent.

Chapter 6: Tinkering with the Future

EPIGRAPH: "11th Chorus" was originally published in *Book of Blues* by Jack Kerouac ©1995, Penguin Poets. Reprinted with the permission of SLL/Sterling Lord Literistic, Inc. Copyright by Jack Kerouac.

1. Implicit in this discussion of Silicon Valley as a crossroad of global flows is Arjun Appadurai's notion of "scapes," in which he discussed five attributes of globalization. These five "building blocks" of the social imaginary are ethnoscapes, mediascapes, technoscapes, finanscapes, and ideoscapes, which describe the movements of people, popular culture, techniques and technologies, capital, ideas, and ideologies (1996, 33).

Bibliography

Albanese, Catherine. *Nature Religion in America: From the Algonkian Indians to the New Age*. Chicago: University of Chicago Press, 1990.

———. *Reconsidering Nature Religion*. Harrisburg, PA: Trinity Press International, 2002.

———. *A Republic of Mind and Spirit: A Cultural History of American Metaphysical Religion*. New Haven: Yale University Press, 2007.

Allen, Tammy D., and Jeremy Armstrong. "Further Examination of the Link between Work-Family Conflict and Physical Health: The Role of Health-Related Behaviors." *American Behavioral Scientist* 49, no. 9 (2006): 1204–21.

Alvarez, Maribel. "There's Nothing Informal about It: Participatory Arts within the Cultural Ecology of Silicon Valley." San José, CA: Cultural Initiatives Silicon Valley, 2005.

Anagnost, Ann. "The Corporeal Politics of Quality (*Suzhi*)." *Public Culture* 16, no. 2 (2004): 189–208.

Aneshensel, Carol S., Amanda L. Botticello, and Noriko Yamamoto-Mitani. "When Caregiving Ends: The Course of Depressive Symptoms after Bereavement." *Journal of Health and Social Behavior* 45, no. 4 (2004): 422–40.

Appadurai, Arjun. *Modernity at Large: Cultural Dimensions of Globalization*. Minneapolis: University of Minnesota Press, 1996.

Arakawa, Hiromu. *Full Metal Alchemist*. Translated by A. Watanabe. San Francisco: VIZ Media, 2002.

Asheim, Bjorn, and Meric Gertler. "The Geography of Innovation: Regional Innovation Systems." In *The Oxford Handbook of Innovation*, edited by Jan

Fagerberg, David Mowery, and Richard Nelson, 291–317. New York: Oxford University Press, 2005.

Auerhahn, Louise, Bob Brownstein, Brian Darrow, and Phaedra Ellis-Lamkins. "Life in the Valley Economy: Silicon Valley Progress Report." San Jose, CA: Working Partnerships USA, 2007, pp. 8–150.

Baba, Marietta. "Dangerous Liaisons: Trust, Distrust, and Information Technology in American Work Organizations." *Human Organization* 58, no. 3 (1999): 331–46.

Baer, Hans. *Biomedicine and Alternative Healing Systems in America: Issues of Class, Race, Ethnicity, and Gender*. Madison: University of Wisconsin Press, 2001a.

———. "The Sociopolitical Status of U.S. Naturopathy at the Dawn of the 21st Century." *Medical Anthropology Quarterly* 15, no. 3 (2001b): 329–46.

———. *Toward an Integrative Medicine: Merging Alternative Therapies with Biomedicine*. Walnut Creek, CA: Altamira Press, 2004.

Banerjee, Payal. "Indian Information Technology Workers in the United States: The H-1b Visa, Flexible Production, and the Racialization of Labor." *Critical Sociology* 32, nos. 2/3 (2006): 425–45.

Barlett, Donald, and Donald Steele. "Critical Condition: How Health Care in America Became Big Business and Bad Medicine." In *The Transformation of Work in the New Economy*, edited by R. Perrucci and C. Perrucci, 593–604. Los Angeles: Roxbury, 2007.

Barley, Stephen, and Gideon Kunda. *Gurus, Hired Guns, and Warm Bodies: Itinerant Experts in a Knowledge Economy*. Princeton: Princeton University Press, 2004.

Barnes, Patricia M., Eve Powell-Griner, Kim McFann, and Richard L. Nahin. "Complementary and Alternative Medicine Use among Adults: United States, 2002." *Advance Data from Vital and Health Statistics* 343 (2004): 1–19.

Baron, James N., Michael T. Hannan, Greta Hsu, and Özgecan Koçak. "In the Company of Women: Gender Inequality and the Logic of Bureaucracy in Start-up Firms." *Work and Occupations* 34, no. 1 (2007): 35–66.

Beck, Ulrich. *Risk Society: Towards a New Modernity*. Thousand Oaks, CA: SAGE Publications, 1992.

Becker, Gay. "Deadly Inequality in the Health Care 'Safety Net': Uninsured Ethnic Minorities' Struggle to Live with Life-Threatening Illnesses." *Medical Anthropology Quarterly* 18, no. 2 (2004): 258–75.

Belasco, Warren. *Meals to Come: A History of the Future of Food.* Berkeley: University of California Press, 2006.

―――. *Appetite for Change: How the Counterculture Took on the Food Industry.* Ithaca, NY: Cornell University Press, 2007.

Belden, Anne. "Virtual Lives: Safety, Time and Relationships: What You Need to Know about Your Child's High-Tech World." *Bay Area Parent,* March 2006, 26–27, 30–31.

Benko, Cathleen, and Anne Weisberg. *Mass Career Customization: Aligning the Workplace with Today's Nontraditional Workforce.* Boston: Harvard Business School Publishing, 2007.

Benner, Chris. *Work in the New Economy: Flexible Labor Markets in Silicon Valley.* Information Age Series. Malden, MA: Blackwell Publishing, 2002.

Bentovim, Orit Avishai. "Family-Friendly as a Double-Edged Sword: Lesson from the 'Lactation-Friendly' Workplace." *Working Paper Series* No. 46, Center for Working Families, University of California, Berkeley, 2002.

Blair, John. *Modular America: Cross-Cultural Perspectives on the Emergence of an American Way.* Westport, CT: Greenwood Press, 1988.

Bookman, Ann. *Starting in Our Own Backyards: How Working Families Can Build Community and Survive the New Economy.* New York: Routledge, 2004.

Bostrom, Nick. "The Transhumanist FAQ: A General Introduction." World Transhumanist Association, http://www.transhumanism.org/resources/FAQv21.pdf (accessed August 2008).

Bourdieu, Pierre. *Outline of a Theory of Practice.* Cambridge, MA: Cambridge University Press, 1977.

―――. *Practical Reason.* Stanford: Stanford University Press, 1998.

Brown, Patricia Leigh. "California Measure Would Align Building Rules with Feng Shui." *New York Times,* January 30, 2004, http://www.nytimes.com/2004/01/30/national/30FENG.html (accessed February 2004).

Buck Consultants. "Empowering Health Consumers." Paper presented at the seventh annual Silicon Valley Conference: The Future of Human Resources, Striking a New Balance. Santa Clara, CA, 2006.

Carey, Pete. "'Long, Slow' Jobs Recovery." *San Jose Mercury News,* November 21, 2009a, A1

―――. "Silicon Valley Jobless Rate Hits 10 Percent for First Time since 1990." *San Jose Mercury News,* March 20, 2009b, C1.

Center for Religious and Civic Culture. "Santa Clara County's Ten Largest Faith Groups in 2000." University of Southern California, http://www.usc.edu/schools/college/crcc/demographics/santaclara.html (accessed April 22, 2008).

Chatterjee, Anjan. "Cosmetic Neurology and Cosmetic Surgery: Parallels, Predictions, and Challenges." *Cambridge Quarterly of Healthcare Ethics* 16 (2007): 129–37.

Chen, Carolyn. "From Filial Piety to Religious Piety: The Immigrant Church Reconstructing Taiwanese Immigrant Families and Parent-Child Relations." Unpublished working paper No. 43. Berkeley, CA: Center for Working Families, 2002.

Chen, Nancy. *Breathing Spaces: Qiqong, Psychiatry and Healing in China*. New York: Columbia University Press, 2003.

Clements, Jonathan, and Helen McCarthy. *The Anime Encyclopedia*. Berkeley: Stone Bridge Press, 2006.

Copeland, Craig. "Labor-Force Participation: The Population Age 55 and Older." *EBRI Notes* 28, no. 6 (2007): 1–10.

Coward, Raymond T., Claydell Horne, and Jeffrey W. Dwyer. "Demographic Perspectives on Gender and Family Caregiving." In *Gender, Families, and Elder Care*, edited by J. W. Dwyer and R. T. Coward, 18–33. Newbury Park, CA: SAGE Publications, 1992.

Cramer, Jeffery S., ed. *Walden: A Fully Annotated Edition*. New Haven: Yale University Press, 2004.

Csordas, Thomas. "Embodiment as a Paradigm for Anthropology." *Ethos* 18, no. 1 (1990): 5–47.

Damasio, Antonio. *Descartes' Error: Emotion, Reason, and the Human Brain*. New York: Grosset/Putnam, 1994.

Darrah, Charles N. "Anthropology and the Workplace-Workforce Mismatch." In *Work, Family, Health and Well-Being*, edited by Suzanne M. Bianchi, Lynne M. Casper, and Rosalind B. King, 201–14. Mahwah, NJ: Lawrence Erlbaum Associates, 2005.

———. "The Anthropology of Busyness." *Human Organization* 66, no. 3 (2007): 261–69.

Darrah, Charles N., James M. Freeman, and J. A. English-Lueck. *Busier than Ever! Why American Families Can't Slow Down*. Stanford: Stanford University Press, 2007.

Darrah, Charles N., Joe Monzel, and Ryan Turner. "Perceptions of Health and Well-Being at San Jose State University." In *Healthy Campus 2010*. San Jose, CA: San José State University, 2007.

de la Rocha, Olivia. "The Reorganization of Arithmetic Practice in the Kitchen." *Anthropology & Education Quarterly* 16, no. 3 (1985): 193–98.

———. "Problems of Sense and Problems of Scale: An Ethnographic Study of Arithmetic in Everyday Life." Dissertation, University of California, Irvine, 1986.

De Natale, Mary Lou. "Understanding the Medicare Part D Prescription Program: Partnerships for Beneficiaries and Health Care Professionals." *Policy, Politics, & Nursing Practice* 8, no. 3 (2007): 170–81.

DeMello, Margo. *Encyclopedia of Adornment*. Westport, CT: Greenwood Press, 2007.

Desai, Prakash. "Health, Faith Traditions, and South Asian Indians in North America." In *Religion and Healing in America*, edited by Linda Barnes and Susan Sered, 423–37. New York: Oxford University Press, 2005.

Dreyer, Danny, and Katherine Dreyer. *Chirunning: A Revolutionary Approach to Effortless, Injury-Free Running*. New York: Fireside, 2004.

Ducharme, Lori, and Jack Martin. "Unrewarding Work, Coworker Support, and Job Satisfaction: A Test of the Buffering Hypothesis." *Work and Occupations* 27, no. 2 (2000): 223–43.

Eisenberg, David M., Roger B. Davis, Susan L. Ettner, Scott Appel, Sonja Wilkey, Maria Van Rompay, and Ronald C. Kessler. "Trends in Alternative Medicine in the United States, 1990–1997: Results of a Follow-up National Survey." *Journal of the American Medical Association* 280, no. 18 (1998): 1569–75.

Elshtain, Jean Bethke. "Toleration, Proselytizing, and the Politics of Recognition." In *Charles Taylor (Philosophy Now)*, edited by Ruth Abby, 127–39. New York: Cambridge University Press, 2004.

English-Lueck, J. A. *Health in the New Age: A Study in California Holistic Practices*. Albuquerque: University of New Mexico Press, 1990.

———. *Cultures@Siliconvalley*. Stanford: Stanford University Press, 2002.

English-Lueck, J. A., Sabrina Valade, Sheri Swiger, and Guillermo Narvaez. "Success and Survival in Silicon Valley." *Educational Outlook* 8, no. 2 (2003): 1–7.

Ezzati, Majid, Ari B. Friedman, Sandeep C. Kulkarni, and Christopher J. L. Murray. "The Reversal of Fortunes: Trends in County Mortality and Cross-

Country Mortality Disparities in the United States." *PLoS Medicine* 5, no. 4 (2008): 1–12.

Falcon, Rod, Marina Gorbis, Lyn Jeffrey, Mani Pande, and J. A. English. "Zones of Instability: A Context for Technology Adoption." In *Technology Horizons Program*. Palo Alto, CA: Institute for the Future, 2006.

Falcon, Rod, and Leah Spalding. "Expanding Meanings of Health." In *Health Horizons Program*. Palo Alto, CA: Institute for the Future, 2004.

Farmer, Paul. *Pathologies of Power: Health, Human Rights, and the New War on the Poor*. Berkeley: University of California Press, 2005.

Farquhar, Judith. *Knowing Practice: The Clinical Encounter of Chinese Medicine*. Boulder, CO: Westview Press, 1994.

———. *Appetites: Food and Sex in Postsocialist China*. Durham, NC: Duke University Press, 2002.

———. "Medicinal Meals." In *Beyond the Body Proper: Reading the Anthropology of Material Life*, edited by Margaret Lock and Judith Farquhar, 287–96. Durham, NC: Duke University Press, 2007.

Farquhar, Judith, and Qicheng Zhang. "Biopolitical Beijing: Pleasure, Sovereignty, and Self-Cultivation in China's Capital." *Cultural Anthropology* 20, no. 3 (2005): 303–27.

Fenstersheib, Marty. "Santa Clara County Health Status Report." San Jose, CA: Public Health Department, Santa Clara Valley Health and Hospital System, 2007.

Ferzacca, Steve. "'Actually, I Don't Feel that Bad': Managing Diabetes and the Clinical Encounter." *Medical Anthropology Quarterly* 14, no. 1 (2000): 28–50.

Finkler, Kaja. "The Healing Genes." In *Religion and Healing in America*, edited by Linda Barnes and Susan Sered, 471–84. New York: Oxford University Press, 2005.

Foehr, Ulla G. "Media Multitasking among American Youth: Prevalence, Predictors and Pairings." Menlo Park, CA: Henry J. Kaiser Family Foundation, 2006.

Fong, Vanessa. "Morality, Cosmopolitanism, or Academic Attainment? Discourses on 'Quality' and Urban Chinese-Only-Children's Claims to Ideal Personhood." *City & Society* 19, no. 1 (2007): 86–113.

Foucault, Michel. *Discipline and Punish: The Birth of the Prison*. Translated by A. Sheridan. New York: Vintage Books, 1995.

Fox, Susannah. "Wired for Health: How Californians Compare to the Rest of the Nation." In *PEW Internet and American Life Project*. Washington, DC: PEW Research Center, 2003.

———. "Generations Online." In *PEW Internet and American Life Project*. Washington, DC: PEW Research Center, 2005.

Fraser, Jill Andresky. "'They Used to Use a Ball and Chain': Technology's Impact on the Workplace." In *The Transformation of Work in the New Economy*, edited by R. Perrucci and C. Perrucci, 140–49. Los Angeles: Roxbury, 2007.

Freeman, James M. *Changing Identities: Vietnamese Americans 1975–1995*. New Immigrant Series, edited by Nancy Foner. Boston: Allyn and Bacon, 1995.

Fuller, Robert. "Subtle Energies and the American Metaphysical Tradition." In *Religion and Healing in America*, edited by Linda Barnes and Susan Sered, 375–85. New York: Oxford University Press, 2005.

Gabe, Jonathan, Mike Bury, and Mary Ann Elston. *Key Concepts in Medical Sociology*. Thousand Oaks, CA: SAGE Publications, 2004.

Gallagher, Shaun. *How the Body Shapes the Mind*. New York: Oxford University Press, 2005.

Galvin, Robert, and Suzanne Delbanco. "Between a Rock and a Hard Place: Understanding the Employer Mind-Set." *Health Affairs* 25, no. 6 (2006): 1548–55.

Gershuny, Jonathan. "Busyness as the Badge of Honor for the New Superordinate Working Class." *Social Research* 72, no. 2 (2005): 287–314.

Gibson, William. *The Science in Science Fiction*. Washington, DC: National Public Radio, 1999.

Giddens, Anthony. *Modernity and Self-Identity: Self and Society in the Late Modern Age*. Stanford: Stanford University Press, 1991.

———. "Risk and Responsibility." *Modern Law Review* 62, no. 1 (1999): 1–10.

Gillis, John. "The Islanding of Children: Reshaping the Mythical Landscapes of Childhood." In *Designing Modern Childhoods: History, Space, and the Material Culture of Children*, edited by Marta Gutman and Ning De Coninck-Smith, 316–30. Piscataway, NJ: Rutgers University Press, 2008.

Gimlin, Debra. *Body Work: Beauty and Self Image in American Culture*. Berkeley: University of California Press, 2002.

Goldfarb, Neil, Christine Weston, Christine W. Hartmann, Mirko Sikirica, Albert Crawford, Hope He, Jamie Howell, Vittorio Maio, Janice Clarke,

Bhaskar Nuthulaganti, and Nicole Cobb. "Impact of Appropriate Pharmaceutical Therapy for Chronic Conditions on Direct Medical Costs and Workplace Productivity: A Review of the Literature." *Disease Management* 7, no. 1 (2004): 61–75.

Goldstein, Michael. *Alternative Health Care: Medicine, Miracle, or Mirage?* Philadelphia: Temple University Press, 1999.

Goodell, Jeff. *Sunnyvale: The Rise and Fall of a Silicon Valley Family.* New York: Villard, 2000.

Google Inc. "Ten Things We Know to Be True." Google Inc., http://www.google.com/intl/en/corporate/tenthings.html (accessed January 15, 2008).

Gorbis, Marina, Rod Falcon, Andrea Tegstam, Anke Schwittay, Lyn Jeffrey, and Bill Cockayne. "Social Networks in the World of Abundant Connectivity." In *Global Innovations Forum*, edited by Charles Grosel and Maureen Davis. Palo Alto, CA: Institute for the Future, 2001.

Hacker, Jacob, ed. *The Great Risk Shift: The Assault on American Jobs, Families, Health Care, and Retirement and How You Can Fight Back.* Rev. and enl. ed. New York: Oxford University Press, 2008.

Haenfler, Ross. *Straight Edge: Cleaning-Living Youth, Hardcore Punk, and Social Change.* New Brunswick, NJ: Rutgers University Press, 2006.

———. *Goths, Gamers, and Grrrls: Deviance and Youth Subcultures.* New York: Oxford University Press, 2010.

Hakken, David. "Computing and Social Change: New Technology and Workplace Transformation, 1980–1990." *Annual Review of Anthropology* 22 (1993): 107–32.

Hall, John, and Charles Lindholm. *Is America Breaking Apart?* Princeton: Princeton University Press, 1999.

Haveman, Heather, and Mukti Khaire. "Organizational Sociology and the Analysis of Work." In *Social Theory at Work*, edited by Marek Korczynski, Randy Hodson, and Paul Edwards, 272–98. New York: Oxford University Press, 2006.

Health Research for Action. "Wellness Priority Area Recommendations for Santa Clara and Northern San Benito County." Campbell, CA: Health Trust, 2007.

Heimer, Carol. "Insurers as Moral Actors." In *Risk and Morality*, edited by Richard V. Ericson and Aaron Doyle, 284–316. Toronto: University of Toronto Press, 2003.

Helman, Ruth, Mathew Greenwald, and Paul Fronstein. "2007 Health Confidence Survey: Rising Health Care Costs Are Changing the Ways Americans Use the Health Care System." *Employee Benefit Research Institute Notes* 28, no. 11 (2007): 1–10.

Helweg, Arthur. *Strangers in a Not-So-Strange Land: Indian American Immigrants in the Global Age*, edited by George Spindler. Case Studies in Cultural Anthropology. Belmont, CA: Wadsworth, 2004.

Henton, Doug. "A Profile of the Valley's Evolving Structure." In *The Silicon Valley Edge: A Habitat for Innovation and Entrepreneurship*, edited by Chong-Moon Lee, William Miller, Hancock Marguerite Gong, and Henry Rowen, 46–58. Stanford: Stanford University Press, 2000.

Henton, Doug, John Melville, Erica Bjornsson, Angelina Aguirre, and Heidi Young. *Index of Silicon Valley*. San Jose, CA: Joint Venture Silicon Valley, 2006.

Henton, Doug, John Melville, Liz Brown, Erica Bjornsson, and Heidi Young. *Index of Silicon Valley*. San Jose, CA: Joint Venture Silicon Valley, 2005.

Henton, Doug, John Melville, Tracey Grose, Angelina Aguirre, Bridget Gibbons, and Hope Ebangi. *Index of Silicon Valley*. San Jose, CA: Joint Venture Silicon Valley Network, 2007.

Henton, Doug, John Melville, Tracey Grose, Gabrielle Maor, Tiffany Furrell, Heidi Young, Dean Chuang, Bridget Gibbons, and Hope Verhulp. *Index of Silicon Valley*. San Jose: Joint Venture Silicon Valley Network, 2009.

Henton, Doug, John Melville, Tracey Grose, Gabrielle Maor, Heidi Young, Bridget Gibbons, and Hope Verhulp. *Index of Silicon Valley*. San Jose: Joint Venture Silicon Valley Network, 2008.

Herzfeld, Michael. *Anthropology: Theoretical Practice in Culture and Society*. Malden, MA: Blackwell Publishers, 2001.

Hess, David. "Crosscurrents: Social Movements and the Anthropology of Science and Technology." *American Anthropologist* 109, no. 3 (2007): 463–72.

Hewlett-Packard. "Rebuilding HP's Garage." Hewlett-Packard Development Company, http://www.hp.com/hpinfo/abouthp/histnfacts/garage/, (accessed March 27, 2008).

Hirschman, Charles "Immigration and the American Century." *Demography* 42, no. 4 (2005): 595–620.

Ho, Evelyn Y. "'Have You Seen Your Aura Lately?' Examining Boundary-Work in Holistic Health Pamphlets." *Qualitative Health Research* 17, no. 1 (2007): 26–37.

Hogle, Linda. "Enhancement Technologies and the Body." *Annual Review of Anthropology* 34 (2005): 695–712.

Horst, Heather, and Daniel Miller. *The Cell Phone: An Anthropology of Communication*. New York: Berg Publishers, 2006.

Hull, Dana. "Autism Expert Shares Life Story as Illustration: Light Shed on Sensory Disorder." *San Jose Mercury News*, September 26, 2004, B1.

Hunt, Alan. "Risk and Moralization in Everyday Life." In *Risk and Morality*, edited by Richard V. Ericson and Aaron Doyle, 165–92. Toronto: University of Toronto Press, 2003.

Hymel, Pamela. "Cisco Systems." Paper presented at the seventh annual Silicon Valley Conference: The Future of Human Resources, Striking a New Balance. Santa Clara, CA 2006a.

———. "Shifting the Focus from Cost to Value: An Employer Perspective." *Journal of Managed Care Pharmacy* 12, no. 6, Supplement B (2006b): S6–10.

Insight Center for Community Economic Development. "Elders Who Can't Make Ends Meet in Santa Clara County as Measured by the California Elder Economic Security Standard Index." Los Angeles: University of California Los Angeles Center for Health Policy Research and the Insight Center for Community Economic Development, 2009.

Ito, Mimi. "Networked Publics: Introduction." http://www.itofisher.com/mito/publications/networked_publi.html (accessed April 24, 2008).

Ito, Mimi, and Heather Horst. "Neopoints, and Neo Economies: Emergent Regimes of Value in Kids Peer-to-Peer Networks." Paper presented at the American Anthropological Association Annual Meetings, San Jose, 2006.

Jackendoff, Ray. *Languages of the Mind: Essays on Mental Representation*. A Bradford Book. Cambridge: MIT Press, 1996.

James, Allison, and Jenny Hockey. *Embodying Health Identities*. New York: Palgrave, 2007.

James, Jack. *Understanding Caffeine: A Behavioral Analysis*. Thousand Oaks, CA: SAGE Publications, 1997.

Jarvis, Helen, and Andy Pratt. "Bringing It All Back Home: The Extensification and 'Overflowing' of Work." *Geoforum* 37, no. 3 (2006): 331–39.

Johanson, Bob. *Get There Early: Sensing the Future to Compete in the Present*. San Francisco: Berrett-Koehler, 2007.

Johnson, Jerry Allen. "Temple of the Celestial Cloud." Tian Yun Gong Zheng

Yi Daoist Temple, http://www.daoistmagic.com/info.php?i=2125 (accessed May 20, 2008).

Johnson, Richard W. "Health Insurance Coverage and Costs at Older Ages: Evidence from the Health and Retirement Study." Washington, DC: AARP, 2006.

Kaptchuk, J., and David Eisenberg. "Varieties of Healing. 2: A Taxonomy of Unconventional Healing Practices." *Annals of Internal Medicine* 135, no. 3 (2001): 196–204.

Karasek, Robert. *Healthy Work: Stress, Productivity and the Reconstruction of Working Life*. New York: Basic Books, 1990.

Kato, Donna. "Baby Steps in Plastic Surgery Are Taken Earlier in Adulthood." *San Jose Mercury News*, July 4, 2004, H1.

Kaufman, Sharon. *And a Time to Die: How Hospitals Shape the End of Life*. New York: Scribner, 2005.

Kaufman, Sharon R., Ann J. Russ, and Janet K. Shim. "Aged Bodies and Kinship Matters: The Ethical Field of Kidney Transplant." *American Ethnologist* 33, no. 1 (2006): 81–99.

Kerouac, Jack. *Book of Blues*. New York: Penguin Poets, 1995.

Kirk, Andrew G. *Counterculture Green: The Whole Earth Catalog and American Environmentalism*. Lawrence: University of Kansas Press, 2007.

Kirsch, Susannah, and Lyn Jeffery. "Boomers in Transition: The Future of Aging and Health." In *Health Horizons Program*. Palo Alto, CA: Institute for the Future, 2003.

Kleinman, Arthur. *The Illness Narratives: Suffering, Healing, and the Human Condition*. New York: Basic Books, 1988.

Kleinman, Arthur, and Joan Kleinman. "Somatization: The Interconnection in Chinese Society among Culture, Depressive Experiences, and the Meanings of Pain." In *Beyond the Body Proper: Reading the Anthropology of Material Life*, edited by Margaret Lock and Judith Farquhar, 468–74. Durham, NC: Duke University Press, 2007.

Kroll-Smith, Steve, and H. Hugh Floyd. *Bodies in Protest: Environmental Illness and the Struggle over Medical Knowledge*. New York: New York University Press, 1997.

Kunitz, Stephen. *The Health of Populations: General Theories and Particular Realities*. New York: Oxford University Press, 2007.

Kuriyama, Shigehisa. "Pulse Diagnosis in the Greek and Chinese Traditions." In *Beyond the Body Proper: Reading the Anthropology of Material Life*, edited by Margaret Lock and Judith Farquhar, 595–607. Durham, NC: Duke University Press, 2007.

Latour, Bruno. "Do You Believe in Reality?" In *Beyond the Body Proper: Reading the Anthropology of Material Life*, edited by Margaret Lock and Judith Farquhar, 176–84. Durham, NC: Duke University Press, 2007.

Lau, Kimberly. *New Age Capitalism: Making Money East of Eden*. Philadelphia: University of Pennsylvania Press, 2000.

Lave, Jean. "The Savagery of the Domestic Mind." In *Naked Science: Anthropological Inquiry in Boundaries, Power, and Knowledge*, edited by L. Nader, 87–100. New York: Routledge, 1996.

Lee, Chong-Moon, William Miller, Hancock Marguerite Gong, and Henry Rowen, eds. *The Silicon Valley Edge: A Habitat for Innovation and Entrepreneurship*. Stanford: Stanford University Press, 2000.

Lenhart, Amanda, Mary Madden, and Paul Hitlin. "Teens and Technology." In *PEW Internet and American Life Project*. Washington, DC: PEW Research Center, 2005.

Lenhart, Amanda, Mary Madden, Alexandra Rankin Macgill, and Aaron Smith. "Teen Content Creators." PEW Research Center, 2007, http://pewresearch.org/pubs/670/teen-content-creators (accessed April 23, 2008).

Lenhart, Amanda, Aaron Smith, Alexandra Rankin Macgill, and Sousan Arafeh. "Writing, Technology and Teens." In *PEW Internet & American Life Project*. Washington, DC: PEW Research Center, 2008.

LeVeen, Emily. "Health Doesn't Just Happen: The Time Crunch and Middle-Class Working Mothers' Use of Complementary and Alternative Medicine." MARIAL Center, 2002, http://www.marial.emory.edu/pdfs/wp018_02.pdf (accessed March 2008).

Levine, Robert. "A Geography of Busyness." *Social Research* 72, no. 2 (2005): 355–70.

Levitin, Daniel. *This Is Your Brain on Music: The Science of a Human Obsession*. New York: Plume, 2006.

Lipson, Juliene G. "Multiple Chemical Sensitivities: Stigma and Social Experiences." *Medical Anthropology Quarterly* 18, no. 2 (2004): 200–13.

Lock, Margaret. "Cultivating the Body: Anthropology and Epistemologies of

Bodily Practice and Knowledge." *Annual Review of Anthropology* 22 (1993): 133–55.

Lock, Margaret, and Judith Farquhar. *Beyond the Body Proper: Reading the Anthropology of Material Life*, edited by Margaret Lock and Judith Farquhar. Durham, NC: Duke University Press, 2007.

Lugo, Luis, Sandra Stencel, John Green, Gregory Smith, Dan Cox, Allison Pond, Tracy Miller, Elizabeth Podrebarac, and Michelle Ralston. "U.S. Religious Landscape Survey." In *PEW Forum on Religion and Public Life*. Washington, DC: PEW Research Center, 2008.

Lyons, Julie Sevrens. "Silicon Valley Life Expectancy Has Jumped from 72 to 80 since 1961." *San Jose Mercury News*, April 22, 2008, http://www.mercurynews.com/Archivesearch (accessed April 2008).

MacEachen, Ellen, Jessica Polzer, and Judy Clarke. "'You Are Free to Set Your Own Hours': Governing Worker Productivity and Health through Flexibility and Resilience." *Social Science & Medicine* 66, no. 5 (2008): 1019–33.

Maher, Brendan. "Poll Results: Look Who's Doping." *Nature* 452 (April 10, 2008): 674–75.

Malone, Thomas. *The Future of Work: How the New Order of Business Will Shape Your Organization, Your Management Style and Your Life*. Boston: Harvard Business School Publishing, 2004.

Markoff, John. *What the Dormouse Said: How the Sixties Counterculture Shaped the Personal Computer Industry*. New York: Penguin, 2006.

Martin, Emily. *Flexible Bodies: Tracking Immunity in American Culture from the Days of Polio to the Age of Aids*. Boston: Beacon Press, 1994.

———. *Bipolar Expeditions: Mania and Depression in American Culture*. Princeton: Princeton University Press, 2007.

Masters, James. "Moksha-Patamu (Snakes and Ladders)." In *The Online Guide to Traditional Games*. Masters Traditional Game Shop, 1997, http://www.tradgames.org.uk/games/Moksha-Patamu.htm (accessed August 2008).

Matthews, Glenna. *Silicon Valley, Women, and the California Dream: Gender, Class and Opportunity in the Twentieth Century*. Stanford: Stanford University Press, 2003.

McAllister, Sue, and Pete Carey. "Santa Clara County Apartment Rents Plunge." *Mercurynews.com*, August 21, 2009, http://www.mercurynews.com/archive-search (accessed December 28, 2009).

McCabe, Sean E., Brady T. West, Michele Morales, James A. Cranford, and Carol J. Boyd. "Does Early Onset of Non-Medical Use of Prescription Drugs Predict Subsequent Prescription Drug Abuse and Dependence? Results from a National Study." *Addiction* 102, no. 12 (2007): 1920–30.

McCabe, Sean E., Christian J. Teter, and Carol J. Boyd. "Medical Use, Illicit Use, and Diversion of Abusable Prescription Drugs." *Journal of American College Health* 54, no. 5 (2006): 269–78.

McCrea, Frances. "The Politics of Menopause: The 'Discovery' of a Deficiency Disease." In *Social Problems across the Life Course*, edited by Helena Lopata and Judith Levy, 227–42. Boulder, CO: Rowman and Littlefield, 2003.

McDonough, William, and Michael Braungart. *Cradle to Cradle: Remaking the Way We Make Things*. New York: North Point Press, 2002.

McEnery, Tom. *The New City-State: Change and Renewal in America's Cities*. Niwot, CO: Roberts Rinehart, 1994.

Mears, Daniel P., and Christopher G. Ellison. "Who Buys New Age Materials? Exploring Sociodemographic, Religious, Network, and Contextual Correlates of New Age Consumption." *Sociology of Religion* 61, no. 3 (2000): 289–313.

Melton, Ginger. "Vying for Power: Gender, Race and Conflict within a High-Technology Corporation." Dissertation, University of Colorado, 2003.

Mennino, Sue Falter, Beth Rubin, and April Brayfield. "Home-to-Job and Job-to-Home Spillover: The Impact of Company Policies and Workplace Culture." In *The Transformation of Work in the New Economy*, edited by R. Perrucci and C. Perrucci, 483–505. Los Angeles: Roxbury, 2007.

Mercury News Wire Services. "Medicine Abuse on Rise among State's Students." *San Jose Mercury News*, October 5, 2006, B5.

Middaugh, Donna. "Presenteeism: Sick and Tired at Work." *MEDSURG Nursing* 15 (2006): 103–5.

Miller, Peter, and Nikolas Rose. *Governing the Present*. Malden, MA: Polity Press, 2008.

Mitchell, Kenneth. "Managing the Corporate Work-Health Culture." *Compensation & Benefits Review* 36, no. 6 (2004): 33–39.

Mizrach, Steve. "Iterative Discourse and the Formation of New Subcultures." *Anthropology of Consciousness* 8, no. 4 (1997): 133–43.

Moen, Phyllis, and Patricia Roehling. *The Career Mystique: Cracks in the American Dream*. Boulder, CO: Rowman and Littlefield, 2005.

Moos, Terry Timm. "National Business Group on Health Honors Best Employers for Healthy Lifestyles." *News@Cisco*, 2007, http://newsroom.cisco.com/dlls/2007/ts_052907.html (accessed March 2008).

Moriarty, Pia. "Immigrant Participatory Arts: An Insight into Community-Building in Silicon Valley." San José, CA: Cultural Initiatives Silicon Valley, 2004.

Murphy, Rachel. "Citizens 'Population Quality' Discourse, Demographic Transition and Primary Education." *China Quarterly* 177 (2004): 1–20.

Napier, Susan. *Anime from Akira to Howl's Moving Castle*. New York: Palgrave, 2005.

Nestle, Marion. *Food Politics: How the Food Industry Influences Nutrition and Health*. Berkeley: University of California Press, 2002.

Nichter, Mark, and Margaret Lock. "Introduction: From Documenting Medical Pluralism to Critical Interpretations of Globalized Health Knowledge, Policies and Practices." In *New Horizons in Medical Anthropology: Essays in Honor of Charles Leslie*, edited by Mark Nichter and Margaret Lock, 1–27. New York: Routledge, 2002.

Novak, Scott, Larry Kroutil, Rick Williams, and David Van Brunt. "The Nonmedical Use of Prescription ADHD Medications: Results from a National Internet Panel." *Substance Abuse Treatment, Prevention, and Policy* 2 (2007): 32–49.

Numbers, Ronald. "The Third Party." In *Sickness and Health in America: Readings in the History of Medicine and Public Health*, edited by J. Leavitt and R. Numbers, 269–83. Madison: University of Wisconsin Press, 1997.

O'Hara, Valerie. *Wellness 9 to 5: Managing Stress at Work*. New York: MJF Books, 1995.

Orta, Andrew. "Syncretic Subjects and Body Politics: Doubleness, Personhood, and Aymara Catechists." *American Ethnologist* 26, no. 4 (2000): 864–89.

Ortner, Sherry B. "Generation X: Anthropology in a Media-Saturated World." *Cultural Anthropology* 13, no. 3 (1998): 414–40.

Park, Lisa Sun-Hee, and David Naguib Pellow. "Racial Formation, Environmental Racism, and the Emergence of Silicon Valley." *Ethnicities* 4, no. 3 (2004): 403–24.

Patel, Julie. "Prescription Stimulant Abused by Some Students Anxious for Edge." *San Jose Mercury News*, May 8, 2005, A1.

Pearlin, Leonard I., Scott Schieman, Elena M. Fazio, and Stephen C. Meersman.

"Stress, Health, and the Life Course: Some Conceptual Perspectives." *Journal of Health and Social Behavior* 46, no. 2 (2005): 205–19.

Pellow, David Naguib, and Lisa Sun-Hee Park. *The Silicon Valley of Dreams: Environmental Injustice, Immigrant Workers, and the High-Tech Global Economy*. New York: New York University Press, 2002.

Pitt-Catsouphes, Marcie. "Work-Friendly or Family Friendly: An Interview with Phyllis Moen and Patricia Roehling, Authors of *The Career Mystique*." Sloan Work and Family Research Network. *Network News* 7, no. 1 (2005): 1–5.

Pitti, Stephen. *The Devil in Silicon Valley: Northern California, Race, and Mexican Americans*. Princeton: Princeton University Press, 2003.

Poletti, Therese. "IBM Settles 50 Lawsuits by Former S.J. Plant Workers: No Terms Were Disclosed in Toxic Chemicals Cases." *San Jose Mercury News*, June 24, 2004, C1.

Public Policy Institute of California. "Dynamics of the Silicon Valley Economy, Just the Facts." San Francisco, CA: Public Policy Institute of California, 2004.

Rafter, Kevin, and Carol Silverman. "Silicon Valley's Changing Nonprofit Sector." In *Regional Nonprofit Sector Report Series*. San Francisco, CA: Institute for Nonprofit Organization Management, University of San Francisco, 2006.

Rainie, Lee. "'Digital Natives' Invade the Workplace." In *PEW Internet and American Life Project*. Washington, DC: PEW Research Center, 2006.

Ramirez, Renya. *Native Hubs: Culture, Community, and Belonging in Silicon Valley and Beyond*. Durham, NC: Duke University Press, 2007.

Rattan, Suresh I. S., and Brian F. C. Clark. "Understanding and Modulating Aging." *IUBMB Life* 57, no. 4/5 (2005): 297–304.

Read, Madlen. "Adults Using Childhood Drugs in Workplace: Treatment Still Needed for Attention Deficit." *San Jose Mercury News*, May 15, 2005, F1.

Redhead, Mark. "Theory and Praxis of Deep Diversity: A Study of the Politics and Thought of Charles Taylor." Dissertation, New School of Social Research, 1999.

———. *Charles Taylor: Thinking and Living Deep Diversity*. Lanham, MD: Rowman and Littlefield, 2002a.

———. "Making the Past Useful for a Pluralistic Present: Taylor, Arendt, and a Problem for Historical Reasoning." *American Journal of Political Science* 46, no. 4 (2002b): 803–18.

Reed-Danahay, Deborah. *Locating Bourdieu*. Bloomington: Indiana University Press, 2005.

Reid, T. R. "Caffeine." *National Geographic* 207, no. 1 (2005): 3–32.

Reischer, Erica, and Kathryn Koo. "The Body Beautiful: Symbolism and Agency in the Social World." *Annual Review of Anthropology* 33 (2004): 297–317.

Reuters Health. "Cognition-Enhancing Drugs Common among Academics." Reuters, http://www.reuters.com/article/healthNews/idUS-TON97705920080409 (accessed April 15, 2008).

Reyes, Belinda, and Jennifer Cheng. "A Portrait of Race and Ethnicity in California: An Assessment of Social and Economic Well-Being." San Francisco, CA: Public Policy Institute of California, 2001.

Robinson, John, and Geoffrey Godbey. "Busyness as Usual." *Social Research* 72, no. 2 (2005): 407–26.

Rose, Nikolas. *The Politics of Life Itself: Biomedicine, Power, and Subjectivity in the Twenty-First Century*. Princeton: Princeton University Press, 2007.

Roszak, Theodore. *Longevity Revolution as Boomers Become Elders*. Berkeley, CA: Berkeley Hills, 2001.

Safe Food International. "Safe Food International." Center for Science in the Public Interest, http://safefoodinternational.org/mission.html (accessed March 2008).

Sangren, P. Steven. "'Power' against Ideology: A Critique of Foucaultian Usage." *Cultural Anthropology* 10, no. 1 (1995): 3–40.

Sauer, Jennifer. "Employment Planning for an Aging Workforce Results from an Aarp California Survey of Employers." Washington, DC: AARP, 2007.

Saxenian, AnnaLee. *The New Argonauts: Regional Advantage in a Global Economy*. Cambridge: Harvard University Press, 2006.

Scheper-Hughes, Nancy. "Nervoso." In *Beyond the Body Proper: Reading the Anthropology of Material Life*, edited by Margaret Lock and Judith Farquhar, 459–67. Durham, NC: Duke University Press, 2007.

Schoenberg, Nancy E., Elaine M. Drew, Eleanor Palo Stroller, and Cary S. Kart. "Situating Stress: Lessons from Lay Discourses on Diabetes." *Medical Anthropology Quarterly* 19, no. 2 (2005): 171–93.

Seipel, Tracy. "Unable to Connect with the World: Asperger's Syndrome Affects Social Skills." *San Jose Mercury News*, June 9, 2002, A16.

Shankar, Shalini. "Windows of Opportunity: South Asian American Teenagers and the Promise of Technology in Silicon Valley." Dissertation, New York University, 2003.

Sharone, Ofer. "Engineering Consent: Overwork and Anxiety at a High-Tech Firm." Unpublished working paper No. 36. Berkeley: Center for Working Families, 2002.

Shih, Johanna. "Project Time in Silicon Valley." *Qualitative Sociology* 27, no. 2 (2004): 223–45.

———. "Circumventing Discrimination: Gender and Ethnic Strategies in Silicon Valley." *Gender and Society* 20, no. 2 (2006): 177–206.

Shore, Bradd. *Culture in Mind: Cognition, Culture, and the Problem of Meaning.* New York: Oxford University Press, 1996.

Siklos, Susan, and Kimberly Kerns. "Assessing Multitasking in Children with ADHD Using a Modified Six Elements Test." *Archives of Clinical Neuropsychology* 19, no. 3 (2004): 347–61.

Silberman, Steve. "We're Teen, We're Queer, and We've Got E-Mail." In *Composing Cyberspace: Identity, Community and Knowledge in the Electronic Age,* edited by Richard Holeton, 116–20. San Francisco: McGraw-Hill, 1998.

———. "The Geek Syndrome." *Wired* 9, no. 12 (2001), http://www.wired.com/wired/archive/9.12/aspergers.html (accessed May 1, 2008).

Silicon Valley Toxics Coalition. "Homepage." Silicon Valley Toxics Coalition, http://www.etoxics.org/site/PageServer (accessed March 2008).

Smola, Karen Wey, and Charlotte Sutton. "Generational Differences: Revisiting Generational Work Values for the New Millennium." *Journal of Organizational Behavior* 23, no. 4 (2002): 363–82.

Snyder, Gary. *Axe Handles: Poems.* San Francisco: North Point Press, 1983.

———. *Danger on Peaks: Poems.* Berkeley: Shoemaker Hoard, 2004.

Starr, Kevin. *California: A History.* New York: Modern Library Chronicles, 2005.

Stern, Lynn. "Public Faces, Private Lives: Making Visible Silicon Valley's Hybrid Heritage Case Study: Macla/Movimiento De Arte Y Cultura Latino Americana." *Animating Democracy E-news* January (2005): 1–15, http://www.americansforthearts.org/animatingdemocracy/pdf/labs/macla_case_study.pdf (accessed April 20, 2008).

Sullivan, Sherry E. "The Changing Nature of Careers: A Review and Research Agenda." *Journal of Management* 25, no. 3 (1999): 457–84.

Sussman, Steve, Mary Ann Pentz, Donna Spruijt-Metz, and Toby Miller. "Misuse of 'Study Drugs': Prevalence, Consequences, and Implications for Policy." *Substance Abuse Treatment, Prevention and Policy* 1 (2006): 15–21.

Swift, Mike. "Boomers Leaving Golden State." *San Jose Mercury News*, May 1, 2008, A1.

Taylor, Charles. "Reconciling the Solitudes: Essays on Canadian Federalism and Nationalism." In *Reconciling the Solitudes: Essays on Canadian Federalism and Nationalism*, edited by Guy LaForest. Montreal: McGill-Queen's University Press, 1993.

———. "The Politics of Recognition." In *Multiculturalism: Examining the Politics of Recognition*, edited by Amy Gutmann, 25–74. Ewing, NJ: Princeton University Press, 1994.

Teraguchi, Daniel Hiroyuki. "The 1954 Brown Decision: Fueling the Torch of Liberation for Asian Pacific Americans." *Diversity Digest* 8, no. 2 (2004): 7.

Thompson, Craig J., and Maura Troester. "Consumer Value Systems in the Age of Postmodern Fragmentation: The Case of the Natural Health Microculture." *Journal of Consumer Research* 28, no. 4 (2002): 550–71.

Tinsley, Barbara. "Multiple Influences on the Acquisition and Socialization of Children's Health Attitudes and Behaviors: An Integrative Review." *Child Development* 63, no. 5 (1992): 1043–69.

Tomes, Nancy. "The Private Side of Public Health: Sanitary Science, Domestic Hygiene, and the Germ Theory, 1870–1900." In *Sickness and Health in America: Readings in the History of Medicine and Public Health*, edited by J. Leavitt and R. Numbers, 506–28. Madison: University of Wisconsin Press, 1997.

Tsing, Anna Lowenhaupt. *Friction: An Ethnography of Global Connection.* Princeton: Princeton University Press, 2005.

Turner, Fred. *From Counterculture to Cyberculture: Stewart Brand, the Whole Earth Network, and the Rise of Digital Utopianism.* Chicago: University of Chicago Press, 2006.

U.S. Census Bureau. "Table 54. Language Spoken at Home—25 Largest Cities: 2005." Washington, DC: U.S. Census Bureau, 2005, http://www.census.gov/compendia/statab/tables/0850054.pdf (accessed March 14, 2008).

———. "Santa Clara County, California Population and Housing Narrative Profile." Washington, DC: U.S. Census Bureau, 2006a, http://factfinder.census.gov/ (accessed March 14, 2008).

———. "United States Population and Housing Narrative Profile." Washington, DC: U.S. Census Bureau, 2006b. Electronic document, http://factfinder.census.gov/ (accessed March 14, 2008).

———. "United States Selected Social Characteristics in the United States." Washington, DC: U.S. Census Bureau, 2006c, http://factfinder.census.gov/ (accessed March 14, 2008).

van Wolputte, Steven. "Hang on to Your Self: Of Bodies, Embodiment, and Selves." *Annual Review of Anthropology* 33 (2004): 251–69.

Varma, Roli. "High-Tech Coolies: Asian Immigrants in the US Science and Engineering Workforce." *Science as Culture* 11, no. 3 (2002): 337–61.

Vian, Kathi, et al. "Boomers, the Next Twenty Years." Palo Alto, CA: Institute for the Future, 2007.

Walters, William. "Later-Life Migration in the United States: A Review of Recent Research." *Journal of Planning Literature* 17, no. 1 (2002): 37–66.

Warner, John Harley. "From Specificity to Universalism in Medical Therapeutics." In *Sickness and Health in America: Readings in the History of Medicine and Public Health*, edited by J. Leavitt and R. Numbers, 87–101. Madison: University of Wisconsin Press, 1997.

Weinberg, Bennett, and Bonnie Bealer. *The World of Caffeine: The Science and Culture of the World's Most Popular Drug.* New York: Routledge, 2001.

Williams, Allan. "Lost in Translation? International Migration, Learning and Knowledge." *Progress in Human Geography* 30, no. 5 (2006): 588–607.

Williams, Florence White. *The Little Red Hen. An Old English Folk Tale.* 1918. Project Gutenberg, 2006, http://www.gutenberg.org/files/18735/18735.txt (accessed December 23, 2009).

Wilson, Nicolas Hoover, and Brian Jacob Lande. "Feeling Capitalism: A Conversation with Arlie Hochschild." *Journal of Consumer Culture* 5, no. 3 (2005): 275–88.

Wong, Bernard. *The Chinese in Silicon Valley: Globalization, Social Networks, and Ethnic Identity.* Boulder, CO: Rowan and Littlefield, 2006.

Yahoo! Inc. "Yahoo! We Value. . . ." Yahoo! Inc., http://docs.yahoo.com/info/values/ (accessed January 15, 2008).

Yan, Hairong. "Neoliberal Governmentality and Neohumanism: Organizing *Suzhi*/Value Flow through Labor Recruitment Networks." *Cultural Anthropology* 18, no. 4 (2003): 493–523.

Zemke, Ron, Claire Raines, and Bob Filipczak. *Generations at Work: Managing the Clash of Veterans, Boomers, Xers, and Nexters in Your Workplace.* New York: AMACOM, 2000.

Zhang, Yanhua. *Transforming Emotions with Chinese Medicine: An Ethnographic Account from Contemporary China.* Albany: State University of New York Press, 2007.

Zissimopoulos, Julie, and Lynn A. Karoly. "Work and Well-Being among the Self-Employed at Older Ages." Washington, DC: AARP, 2007.

Zlolniski, Christian. "Labor Control and Resistance of Mexican Immigrant Janitors in Silicon Valley." *Human Organization* 62, no. 1 (2003): 39–49.

———. *Janitors, Street Vendors, and Activists: The Lives of Mexican Immigrants in Silicon Valley.* Berkeley: University of California Press, 2006.

Index